From SHATTERED *Dreams*

Dorothy R. Ruhwald

My Journey Through Postpartum Psychosis

FROM SHATTERED DREAMS
My Journey Through Postpartum Psychosis

Scripture quotations marked NIV are taken from the Holy Bible, New International Version. Copyright © 1973, 1978, 1984 by International Bible Society. Used by permission of Zondervan Publishing House. Scripture quotations marked NASB are taken from the New American Standard Bible, Copyright © 1960, 1962, 1963, 1971, 1972, 1973, 1975, 1977, 1995 by The Lockman Foundation. Used by permission.

ISBN-13: 978-1-926676-58-6

Printed in Canada.

Printed by Word Alive Press
131 Cordite Road, Winnipeg, MB R3W 1S1
www.wordalivepress.ca

To *The Refiner*, who
shakes everything that can
be shaken, so that what cannot
be shaken may remain.

FOREWORD

Postpartum… a word which brings to mind that period of time when a mother and father's wait is finally over. A time when a new baby is held close and loved, as the proud parents look forward to a new, exciting future, and… psychosis? Certainly that word does not seem to fit with the special time following a baby's birth, when dreams should be coming true. Rather the word psychosis would sooner be connected with a nightmare, striking fear into the very heart of a person. For one in 1,000 new mothers, however, it is a terrifying fact - postpartum psychosis.

Because of the stigma in society regarding mental illness, it can be very difficult for those who have been touched by postpartum psychosis to reach out for support.

Who can they risk talking to? Is there anyone who understands? And that is my main purpose in writing this book – to offer information, support, and encouragement through my own personal experience with postpartum psychosis.

If you or a loved one has experienced postpartum psychosis, I pray that this book will encourage you, and bring you one step closer to healing. If you are involved in the medical profession, especially with mental illness, may you receive a greater understanding, and the ability to look beyond the *symptoms* to the frightened, hurting person, trying so hard to cope. Whatever your reason for reading this book, may you come to a new awareness of the God who takes you *from shattered dreams*, to healing, greater character, and new purpose.

TABLE OF CONTENTS

ONE

A Young Girl's Dream

I walked down the hallway of our apartment and looked almost fearfully into the nursery. Upon entering, I could see the crib complete with the quilt and bumper pads I had sewn just months earlier. Along the opposite wall was the change table filled with tiny diapers, undershirts, and sleepers. Stacked on the floor were baby presents, many of them unopened--but there was something vitally important missing. Where there should have been a tiny baby, filling the room with its sweet presence, there was only a great emptiness. Where there should have sounded the cries of a newborn, there was silence. A silence which threatened to overwhelm me.

When would the silence end? When would I be able to look into that room and find my baby there? These were questions that haunted me. After all, wasn't it because of me there was no baby in the nursery?

I was just now out of hospital, not from the maternity ward, but from the psychiatric ward. My baby had been born two months earlier, and I was home from hospital on my first weekend pass. Although the doctor and nurses all agreed I was much better, the date of my actual release was still uncertain. When that day came, perhaps then I could begin to forget the nightmare I had experienced and glue together the pieces of my dream. My dream...it had all seemed so simple then.

⋏   ⋏   ⋏

Some girls dream of owning a pet, others a Barbie dollhouse. But what I wanted most in life, from the time I was a very young girl, was to have my very own baby. A doll just wasn't good enough; I wanted the real thing.

Many hours were spent leafing through the mail order catalogues, looking at all the sweet little babies. There were such wonderful things to order along with these babies, from miniature dresses and sleepers, to a crib for the baby to sleep in. I could be set up for life. "Daddy, do you think I could have a baby of my very own?" I asked my father one day.

"A baby? Well, we'll have to see... maybe for Christmas," he answered. For Christmas I received a doll, not at all what I was hoping for. It was disappointing to learn that babies could not just be ordered from a catalogue. Now my only hope was that some kind person might leave a baby on my doorstep. It may have happened on TV, but not at my house. Still, the desire to take in children who had no home of their own stayed. I began considering the idea of working in an orphanage. My mother had taught in an orphanage for a short time before her marriage. From her description of that time in her life, one thing really stuck in my mind. Some of the ladies working at the orphanage would bring a few children to their home for the Christmas holidays. To me, that was just great. I would get a job at an orphanage, take a couple of kids home for Christmas and just keep them.

As the years went by, my great idea of adopting a house full of orphans faded. I decided that having a few babies of my own might be a bit more realistic. Since a father was needed for the children, this was added to my future plans as well. I considered going into the field of Early Childhood Education, but when it came down to it, taking care of a husband and children was the only career I really wanted.

From the time my own mother got married, she was a homemaker, and she did it well. I was the fourth child out of five, having two older brothers, an older sister, and one younger brother. Being in a large family was great; there was never a problem finding someone to play with. Mom really made our house into a home. As we would walk in the door after school, there was often the smell of fresh bread or cookies in the air. It wasn't so much the baking, although that sure helped. It was her being there, ready to listen to us if we wanted to talk. It was the time spent together baking Christmas cookies or sewing a dress. All of these things passed on a real sense of love and security--and it was this kind of mother that I wanted to be once I had my own children.

There was one gift I received from Mom which turned out to be far more important than learning to sew or cook; this was demonstrating to me the importance of memorizing Bible verses. I had attended Sunday school and church all my life. Bible memorization was typically a part of that, but Mom encouraged me to take it further. I began to memorize verses on my own, especially during my teen years.

Growing up in a Christian family, I believed that God was ultimately in control of my future. It was only natural to pray about my hopes and dreams, asking God to lead me to the right man: a Christian who would be a good husband and father. There was no doubt in my mind that God had a plan for my life; I just hoped it would match up with mine.

There was this niggling thought in the back of my mind: What if God doesn't want me to get married or have kids? What if He wants me to stay single and become a missionary in some far-off remote place like Africa?

I was really beginning to wonder what God had in mind when, at the great age of sixteen, there was not even a boyfriend in sight. However, there was no need to worry, for shortly thereafter I met my future husband.

I had my first glimpse of Kurt when he walked into our church one Sunday. Being a fairly small church, it wasn't that unusual to have noticed him. The pastor introduced Kurt to my oldest brother Wilfred, who was president of the College and Career group at that time. It turned out that Kurt was a pilot and had just been transferred to my hometown, Prince George. Wilfred and Kurt struck up a friendship and one Sunday he invited Kurt over for lunch. As Kurt and I sat around the dinner table that day, our eyes just happened to meet, more than once. My first impression of Kurt was that he had a very nice smile with especially warm brown eyes. Apparently Kurt had noticed me in church as well and was intrigued that I was Wilfred's sister.

After that day, Kurt would often come over to our house for Sunday dinner, and I learned through Wilfred that he had made some nice comments about me. Well, that started me speculating and dreaming, as teenage girls are inclined to do. Kurt had no idea that I knew what he had said about me. In fact, he was interested in me, but he was concerned about the seven-year age difference between us. It took a few months for him to get over this, during which time I had pretty well given up on him. One Sunday night things began to change. After the church service, I was clearing the snow off the windshield of my car when who should come over to me, but Kurt. "Here, I'll do that for you!" he said, proceeding to brush the snow off my entire car.

I was impressed! What a gentleman! My older brothers often teased me as if I was still a little girl. To be treated like a lady was really special.

Driving home that night, my car seemed to float a few feet off the ground. I tried to remind myself not to get my hopes up. After all, Kurt was probably just being nice. He didn't necessarily mean anything by it. But still, I couldn't help being excited.

A few days later I received my first phone call from Kurt. My brother, Wilfred, laughingly called, "Dorothy, Kurt is on the phone for you!"

"Yah, right," I said. My brother was entirely capable of saying this only to tease me. It was quite a surprise to actually hear Kurt on the phone, and I was even more surprised when he asked me out to a movie. Of course I said yes. Rushing around the house getting ready, there was the sound in the background of Dad singing "I'm Dreaming of a White Christmas," only inserting "nice pilot" for "White Christmas." My parents were evidently excited too. After all, their little girl was going on her first date. For the big event I took a bath and curled my hair, wanting to make the best impression. It was all very exciting but I was also a bit nervous. "What would we talk about?" I wondered. I was really quite shy and didn't want him to think me just a silly school girl.

As it turned out, we had a great time. Some of Kurt's friends met us at the movie theatre, and we all went out for pizza with them afterwards. His friends were very outgoing and funny so I soon felt quite comfortable with them all.

After that night, our relationship progressed rapidly. I started being the one to invite Kurt home for dinner on Sundays. We went night skiing, roller-skating, and talked often on the phone. Somehow we just seemed to fit together. Kurt was very easy for me to talk to, maybe because we came from the same German background and had much the same belief system. From the time we started dating, I never really thought that our relationship might end. It just felt so natural.

That spring, after we had been dating for around four months, Kurt took me to meet his parents in Victoria. One day we went to a beautiful park filled with trees and flowers. We sat down on a bench overlooking a pond, where many ducks were milling around, quacking rather loudly and impatiently waiting to be fed. It was in this romantic setting that Kurt proposed. I didn't need to think twice about saying yes, although I didn't do so lightly. This was a big commitment and my life would never be the same. "Well, this is it," I thought. There's no turning back now. Not that I wanted to turn back. It's just that heading into an unknown future was not only exciting but also rather intimidating. I guess it was like the feeling you get the day after Christmas. It was all very fun and exciting but now what?

Although at seventeen I was still quite young to be thinking of marriage, my parents had no objections, at least none they shared with me. It was what I had always wanted and they couldn't help but approve of Kurt. After all, he met the important criteria: he was a Christian, was able to support me, and he loved me.

Aside from telling our respective parents about our marriage plans, we decided to keep it a secret until my high school graduation. That was a very special night. Not only did I receive a graduation diploma, but from Kurt I received a dozen roses and an engagement ring. We planned to get married the following spring, giving me time to complete an Early Childhood Education program at our community college.

After starting college in the fall, I began to lose a lot of weight and to feel progressively more tired. It didn't dawn on me that I might be ill because my symptoms started so gradually. After visiting the doctor, though, I was diagnosed with Grave's disease, or hyperthyroidism. My thyroid gland was overactive, causing a general speeding-up of all the chemical reactions in my body, mentally as well as physically. At that time, a common treatment for hyperthyroidism was to drink radioactive iodine. This would kill off part of the thyroid gland, hopefully the right amount. I opted to go for this course of treatment so my mother and I headed off to the hospital in Vancouver with Kurt as our chauffeur.

By this time, I was feeling very stressed out. My muscles were weak, my hands and neck were trembly, and I had a dangerously fast and irregular heartbeat (and here I had thought it was Kurt that was making my heart beat so fast)! Emotionally, I was very energetic and excited one minute, then quite depressed the next.

Although I had, in many ways, really enjoyed the courses at the college and was doing quite well, it just seemed too much to handle at that time. Previously I had not even considered quitting college, but during our stay in Vancouver I discussed it with Mom. It was not easy for me to quit almost halfway through the program, but once I decided to actually go ahead and do it, I experienced such a feeling of relief. Now I could go home, relax, and enjoy the remaining time before the wedding.

Within a few months of my iodine treatment, I felt completely well again. Much of my time was spent with

Kurt but I also prepared for married life by practicing my cooking and baking skills.

The wedding was set for June and I did much of the organization myself. Mom and I had great fun baking fancy cakes for the open house which would follow the reception. Our freezer was packed full.

On June 11, 1983, Kurt and I were married. With the ceremony at 1:00 P.M., followed by the reception and open house, it was a very full, if exciting, day. Our wedding night was spent in a hotel, and then the next day we moved into our mobile home. Kurt had only that weekend off; he had to go back to work on Monday. It was a very short honeymoon but with Kurt's job flying in the bush he had to work when he could. Generally the bush flying would happen during the summer, leaving him without work during the winter.

The reality of being a pilot's wife set in very quickly. The first week of our marriage Kurt got stuck out of town for three days due to weather. I had married Kurt knowing that as a pilot he wouldn't be home every night. It did take a bit of getting used to, though. To keep myself from getting lonely, I got involved in the Pioneer Girls program at our church and also in teaching Sunday school. All in all, I really enjoyed married life. It was especially fun making our trailer into a home.

Although it may seem as if I had a real Cinderella complex, I think my expectations of married life were quite realistic. I knew there was no such thing as "happily ever after." I was naive though, thinking that other people might go through financial difficulties, or get sick, but that wouldn't happen to us. As it turned out, we had our share of both in the first few years of marriage.

When Kurt's flying came to an end after that first summer, we were very pleased when he got a job flying for a logging company. It meant up to ten days away from home at a time, but at least it was steady work. Unfortunately, the company expected him to perform duties other than those he was initially hired for. After only two months of work, Kurt injured his back while doing some shovelling. By Christmas Kurt was unable to work; he had ruptured a disc. After bed rest was tried without any success, the doctors decided an operation was necessary. It proved to be unsuccessful as well. Although it was perhaps a risky thing to do, Kurt decided to undergo a second back operation. This time the operation was a success, although there was still a long healing process to go through. Kurt was unable to work for the entire year of 1984.

During that year we had two major questions running through our minds: 1) Would Kurt ever be able to fly again? 2) Would his back ever heal enough so he wouldn't be in constant pain? I knew that for Kurt the biggest dream of *his* life had been to fly and eventually work for an airline.

To lose that dream would be very difficult for him to accept. Besides these questions we also had great concerns about our financial situation. Workers' Compensation was reluctant to believe that Kurt's injury occurred at work. I got a job at a bakery-delicatessen but my wages were hardly enough to support us. It was a very difficult time for us but there was a positive side. Our commitment to each other grew and we were drawn even closer together. We also realized more fully that we were not in control of our lives; God held our future in His hands and we needed to depend on Him.

We took these questions and fears to God and He really answered. Not only did Kurt's back heal amazingly well but also Workers' Compensation came through for us just as our savings were dropping to zero.

I can honestly say that I hoped our hard times would be over, that we would now have an easy life, with no more financial difficulties or illness. We had gone through much in the first two years of our marriage. Now it was time for us to get on with our lives and careers.

When Kurt finally felt well enough to work again, he sent out several resumes to different airlines. In spring of the next year he got hired by a helicopter company. He flew helicopter parts and people all over Northern BC, getting a chance to view some wonderful scenery. Kurt worked for this company for two summers and really enjoyed it. He couldn't help wondering, though, if he would ever get on with a "real scheduled airline" and be able to work the whole year through. So he kept sending those resumes out, hoping that when the airline industry began to expand again, he could get on with a larger airline.

In the meantime we decided to go ahead and start a family. Both my sister and my sister-in-law had babies the previous year; now it was my turn. When I found out that I was pregnant I was ecstatic. My dream was really going to come true. When the morning sickness wore off, I began to happily plan for the baby; I even took up knitting.

Things seemed to be finally picking up for us by the spring of 1987. Not only did we have a baby on the way, but also Kurt was hired by a larger airline, which was rapidly expanding. We couldn't ask for anything more. The job meant a move away from my hometown, Prince George, to the much larger city of Vancouver, BC. Although I knew I would miss my family, the excitement of living on the coast, and the knowledge that our baby would soon arrive, over-shadowed any negative feelings I may have had.

We had a very busy few weeks before our actual move. Kurt had already started working in Vancouver in May. It was left to me to pack up what I could and put our trailer up for sale. In June we packed all of our possessions into a moving truck and headed off to our new home, just in time to celebrate our fourth wedding anniversary in the big city.

TWO

Baby Arrives

Our new home was an apartment in Richmond, a suburb of Vancouver. It was very appropriate for a pilot's family. Not only was it close to the Vancouver airport, meaning a short drive to work for Kurt, but we could watch (and hear) the jets go by right from our balcony.

Because the Vancouver area was such a change from my hometown, I found it very interesting and exciting. On my previous visits to Vancouver the city had seemed very hectic with the heavy traffic and large population. In contrast, living in Richmond was relatively peaceful. I rarely had to drive right into the city of Vancouver and Richmond was much smaller and more manageable. Soon I was able to go for a drive without worrying about finding my way home again.

Kurt was born in Vancouver so he knew all of the fun things to do and neat places to visit. On his days off, we would take a few hours and explore different parks and beaches, go for walks, or fly a kite. We also found that from our home, it was only a few blocks to a dike, where there was a very popular path for walking, running, and cycling. It was just beautiful; we would see ducks, muskrat, and many different kinds of birds. Our home seemed to include the best of both worlds: living in a big city with a piece of country almost right in our backyard.

However, our life wasn't just a holiday. Kurt had his job to do and he was really enjoying it. As co-pilot in a twin otter, he would fly to Vancouver Island and Seattle. It was a challenge learning to fly a new aircraft and adjusting to the many changes involved in flying for a scheduled airline.

Although Kurt would often fly long hours, I was fortunate enough to have him home every night. There was also plenty to keep me occupied while he was working. Aside from unpacking and organizing all of our things in the apartment, I had the new baby to prepare for. I began fixing up the nursery, setting up a crib and change table in our second bedroom. I went on a shopping spree in the fabric store, buying material to make bumper pads and a quilt for

15

the crib, and enough flannel for receiving blankets and wash cloths. If sewing didn't keep me busy enough, I still had my knitting project to work on. Initially, my plan was to knit a tiny dress. It was becoming increasingly clear that my yarn had been much thicker than the pattern had called for. Even as a novice knitter I could see that five feet was a bit much to go around one small baby. Oh, well. Since I refused to give up and pull out my many hours of hard work, we ended up with a blanket instead—a super-sized blanket which the baby could use for many years to come. In fact, right to adulthood.

Kurt and I were both busy, but we tended to be more isolated since our move. There was no dinner at my parents' house every Sunday. It was also not quite as easy to pick up the phone and talk to my family. In one way this was probably beneficial for our relationship. Since we often didn't have others to talk to, we needed to rely more on each other, really becoming "best friends."

Even though none of my immediate family was in the Vancouver area, my Aunt Helen, Uncle Bob, and two cousins—Jason, and Sabrina—lived within walking distance of our home. Kurt also had many relatives in Vancouver and his parents lived in Victoria, which would be only a few hours away if we were to visit.

After settling into our new home, one of my first priorities was to find a good doctor. Aunt Helen recommended her family doctor to me, Dr. Davis. He turned out to be very personable and easy to talk to. I was relieved to find a good doctor so quickly. Because of my history of thyroid problems Dr. Davis also referred me to a gynaecologist in case of any complications during pregnancy and delivery.

Another priority was to find a church. We decided to attend a Baptist church in Vancouver that Kurt had gone to when he was a child. One of the church families, who just happened to also lived in Richmond, invited us to their weekly bible study. This study really helped us to get to know a few families on more than just a surface level.

Between Kurt's job, my work at home, and church activities, the weeks seemed to go by quickly. I was really enjoying my pregnancy. Physically I was feeling great. It was so special to feel the baby move inside me and wonder what he or she would be like. Kurt and I went to prenatal classes, preparing us for the labour and delivery of the baby.

As the due date grew closer, my anticipation to see this new baby grew, but September 17 came and went with still no baby. As the days went by, I almost despaired of ever leaving my pregnant state. Non-stress tests were done repeatedly to make sure the baby was all right, but there were still no signs that he/she was ready to make an appearance any time soon.

On September 26th I had yet another non-stress test. That evening Dr. Davis phoned, explaining, "Dorothy, I think it's time to go for an induction. At this point the baby would be better off delivered. You're not showing any signs that you will go into labour naturally. We'll try inducing you ... if that doesn't work, you may need a Caesarean."

A Caesarean ...! That was something I just hadn't anticipated. I would so much rather have the baby naturally. If there was even a slight possibility of it coming to a Caesarean, though, I wanted to be prepared. I poured through any and all information on Caesarean sections that I had received from my prenatal classes. This knowledge may have equipped me to some extent but I still wasn't thrilled by the idea, so when Kurt arrived home from work, I blurted out, "Dr. Davis says I might need a Caesarean..." and promptly burst into tears.

Sunday evening I was admitted to hospital and prepared to be induced the next day. Apart from some trepidation about the approaching delivery I was really quite excited. Most people don't find staying in the hospital anything to get excited about, but this was a first for me, making it novel and interesting. By this time I had also prepared myself emotionally as best I could for the next day. One way or another, my baby would be born.

Lying in my bed that night I prayed, "God, just give me strength to go through the labour and delivery, whatever happens." I went to sleep thinking about the coming arrival of the baby. I would actually be a mother. My life would definitely change. But I didn't realize that it would change more drastically and in different ways than I had ever dreamed possible.

Early the next morning I was given medication to induce labour. Thankfully the medication did its job, but it was a very slow process. I was practically tied to my bed all day since my contractions and the baby's heartbeat were being continually monitored. Kurt stayed at my side but unfortunately apart from his supportive presence, there wasn't all that much he could do. It would have been nice if he could have taken a turn, and given me a break! I felt that I was going through an endurance test, a long marathon of pains that would hopefully end soon.

By evening I was in hard labour. Our baby was born, naturally, around 10 P.M. She was absolutely beautiful, with great big round eyes and one inch of thick black hair covering her head. We named her Martina Rose. Although the name was chosen months earlier, it certainly suited her. She was a real rose among babies. Eventually we might discover some thorns, but for now she seemed just perfect. Holding Martina, I thought, "Wow! We're truly fortunate to be given such a special baby to care for."

After holding Martina for a few minutes, I passed her on to the proud Daddy. Right away we nicknamed her "Sucker," as she was loudly sucking on her fist, making noises like a little piglet. It was difficult to comprehend that here we had a little person who had up until then been surviving inside of my body. Martina was still part of both of us, yet she had her own little personality.

The birth of the baby had gone very well, and my gynaecologist, Dr. Mackie, felt it unnecessary to stay any longer. He left Dr. Davis to finish up. Within minutes of delivering the placenta, however, I began to haemorrhage profusely. Blood seemed to be everywhere, pumping out with every beat of my heart. It had started so suddenly. We abruptly went from being the "happy parents with new baby" to the focal point in an emergency situation. Dr. Mackie was urgently paged as Dr. Davis frantically tried to find the cause of bleeding.

Numerous thoughts rushed through my mind: "Maybe I'll need a hysterectomy. At least I have one baby... What if I bleed to death? How will Kurt care for the baby by himself?"

I remember looking up at Kurt, who was at my side. His face was pale and I could see the fear in his eyes. Strangely enough, I didn't feel a great deal of fear myself. My concern was more for the baby and Kurt. As I lay there this passage of scripture came to mind:

> "Let not your heart be troubled; believe in God, believe also in Me. In My Father's house are many dwelling places; if it were

not so, I would have told you; for I go to
prepare a place for you. And if I go and prepare a place for you, I will come again, and
receive you to Myself; that where I am, there
you may be also." (John 14:1-3, NASB)

I had always heard of verses coming to people right
when they needed them but in this case I wasn't sure about
God's choice! I liked the part about my heart not being
troubled, but I really didn't want to visit those heavenly
dwelling places just yet. That could, I hoped, wait a few
years. I guess God thought so too. By the time my gynaecologist arrived, Dr. Davis had been able to stop the bleeding. Apparently my cervix had torn. Together the doctors
stitched me up. I was then rolled into the recovery room,
where I was again given baby Martina to hold and to nurse.

After Martina was taken to the nursery for the night,
Kurt dragged himself home to get some sleep. I didn't feel
all that tired myself, just surprisingly weak physically.
When taking out my contacts for the night, it took all my
strength to squeeze the saline solution out of its bottle.
Aside from my weakness, I was in good spirits, very happy
and excited, not to mention thankful that everything had
worked out so well.

Although I had been given some medication to help me
sleep, I lay awake a while thinking about the baby—my very

own baby. I remembered my sister Marie saying: "Having a baby is like getting a wonderful present." Well, that's just how it felt. I was really looking forward to the next morning when I could hold Martina, unwrap her, and begin getting to know this tiny person—this tiny person who had already become so important in my life.

By morning my excitement over the new baby was still there, but it was subdued somewhat by my extreme physical weakness. Two nurses were needed to escort me to the washroom. If I tried to stand up on my own, my vision would go black and I would feel very dizzy. I was also in considerable discomfort. Just rolling over in bed was a chore. Although I was able to hold Martina when feeding her, it was the nurses who changed and bathed her. I should have been grateful to have someone else change her for me—after all, I would have many chances in the months ahead—but somehow I felt cheated. These were things that, as her mother, I felt should be done by me. However, it was obvious that I just was not up to it yet. Between the loss of blood and lack of food the day before, I was completely exhausted.

Later that morning, Dr. Davis decided a blood transfusion was in order. Shortly after it was administered I ate a large lunch, my first meal since arriving in hospital two nights ago. The combination of the transfusion and the meal did wonders for me. I was able to change the baby and walk through the ward on my own. From then on I recovered my strength rapidly.

It took only a few days for me to feel well enough to go home, but Martina had developed jaundice so our hospital stay was extended. Although I was feeling well physically, some insidious changes to my personality began to emerge. I began to feel euphoric. There was a growing excitement inside of me, as if in anticipation of something special about to happen in my life. Although I was normally quite shy, I was suddenly outgoing, talking much more than usual with the women who shared my room in hospital. They were total strangers, yet it seemed as if I had known them all of my life.

The thought crossed my mind that since having a baby made me feel so wonderful I would like to have many more. Forgotten were the crisis events of the preceding days. Forgotten was anything at all negative. The world was a fantastic place to live in. To say I was seeing the world through rose coloured glasses would be an understatement.

Although these daytime thoughts all seemed very positive, I had two dreams one night, which were just the opposite. They were really quite silly in and of themselves. In the first dream I saw some peculiar jelly-like bugs on the wall. In the second dream a mentally handicapped person, who appeared very afraid, ran into a bathroom and jumped onto the back of the toilet tank. Someone ran after him, trying to reassure him and get him down. I woke from both of these dreams with a start, feeling a fear deep inside of me. In all my life I have never had a dream that affected me in quite that way. These dreams disturbed me, but I didn't really give them too much lingering thought. I concluded that I was probably just overtired from feeding Martina during the night.

It was certainly true that I had good reason to be over-tired. Martina seemed to be going through a growth spurt, wanting to nurse often, and for long periods during the night. I wasn't getting much sleep, yet I didn't feel tired. I actually felt hyperactive and energetic—and unusually hungry. The hospital food tasted great to me but there just wasn't enough of it. I made frequent trips to the kitchen for food or for something to drink; I even got Kurt to bring me food from home on his visits. On one nocturnal trip to the kitchen for a drink, I walked around a corner and almost bumped into a nurse. Strange that this chance encounter should make me jump like I did. I felt like my nerves were stretched unbearably tight, making me not only very edgy, but also jumpy.

By the weekend, Martina's jaundice was improving. Dr. Davis felt we could be released shortly, so Mom flew to Vancouver to help me with the baby. When her flight arrived, Kurt brought her to the hospital to visit me. As soon as she walked through my door I gave her a big hug. This was rather unusual behaviour for me, because although I had a great relationship with Mom, the members of our family didn't often show physical affection so freely. It wasn't even so much giving Mom a hug that was unusual; I may have done that anyway. Rather it was how I felt about giving the hug—very open, natural, and self-confident. It was as though any inhibitions I may have had were disappearing.

Mom had brought with her a huge box of used baby clothes from my sister Marie, and several presents. It was better than Christmas rooting through everything, and checking what items would fit Martina. She would definitely not be short of things to wear; Marie had even handmade her some adorable berets with little airplanes on them.

During this visit and every other time Mom came, I talked fast and furiously; there just seemed to be so much to say. This change in me didn't go completely unnoticed by Mom. It was quite obvious to her that I was having a "mountain-top" experience, but she thought that reality would settle in soon enough.

Finally we were ready to be released from hospital. One week after Martina was born, on Monday, Oct. 5th, we prepared to go home. Martina, in her new car seat, was securely strapped into the car, and off we went. Although it was October, the weather outside was sunny and warm, matching my own feelings inside. I was looking forward, with great anticipation, to my new role as a mother.

THREE

From a Dream to a Nightmare

*I*t was great to finally get home, away from the noise and activity of the hospital. With Mom on hand to help out, I was looking forward to a relaxing time of just visiting and caring for the baby. Martina seemed happy to be home as well; after being fed and changed she settled quite contentedly into her crib for a nap.

Mom urged me to take the opportunity and have a rest myself. I lay down on my bed for only a few minutes. I just wasn't feeling tired. There was too much on my mind to consider sleeping. I felt as if my head was crowded with thoughts and ideas, all wanting to be expressed. I used my mother as a sounding board, talking almost nonstop. My mind couldn't seem to manage shaping so many ideas into words at such a great speed, however. I would be talking away in a steady stream when suddenly my mind would go blank, causing me to completely forget what I had been saying. That was not enough to stop me—there was always something else equally important, at least in my mind, which needed to be said.

I finally took a break from talking when Martina awoke from her nap. After feeding her, I dressed her up for the evening. We were all invited over to my Aunt Helen and Uncle Bob's place for supper. This would be Martina's first official outing and I wanted her to look really special. I tried on many different outfits, finally settling on a flowery blue dress with lace trim, and for the perfect finishing touch, a matching airplane beret.

The dinner went well; for a change I was relatively quiet. I wanted to give Mom a chance to visit with her sister. After dinner Kurt went to a meeting at work, leaving us to stay until he came to pick us up later that evening. As Mom and Aunt Helen talked, I laid Martina on the living room floor, watching closely as Sabrina "played" with her. Even though I was not talking much, I had an inner awareness that something was different, a feeling of mental alertness and well being.

Martina had been very happy and content throughout the whole visit, but by the time Kurt picked us up to go home she was expressing her displeasure rather loudly. She screamed all the way home, which I found very upsetting, but after being fed she went right off to sleep. I settled down to sleep as well, but not for long. Martina didn't know the meaning of sleeping through the night; she generally ate every three or four hours. When Martina awoke I changed her, and then nursed her in the living room so I wouldn't wake Mom, who was sharing the nursery with the baby. After feeding Martina I quietly slipped into the nursery and laid her back down in the crib. Mom was awake, if only slightly. I took this as an invitation to begin talking again: "You know Mom, I feel as if all of my senses are so much more sharp and aware since I had the baby. My hearing, sight, and even my brain seem to be at maximum power..." and on I went. An hour later I finally went back to bed.

Martina was up for another feeding at 4 A.M. Kurt was having his breakfast at that time as well; he had an early shift of flying that day. After he left I went back to bed, sleeping until around seven o'clock. As I lay in bed after waking I had a very strange sensation. It felt as if my whole bedroom flipped right over. I quickly got out of bed—the ground seemed to be moving under my feet!

I ran into the baby's room calling, "Mom, did you feel the earthquake?"

"Earthquake?" Mom sleepily answered. "Dorothy, are you sure? I didn't feel a thing."

"You can't feel it? The ground is moving!" As I stood there the ground seemed to be undulating. "Richmond is all built on peat moss. I guess that's why it feels like this." As Mom got out of bed I laughed and said, "See, you're even walking funny!"

Mom was not at all convinced that there had been an earthquake but for her to persuade me otherwise was also impossible. I had definitely felt something; if Mom didn't, that didn't make it any less real to me. When the "earthquake" was over I went to take a shower and get ready for the day.

Our plans for the day included some grocery shopping. Since Kurt had our only vehicle at work, Aunt Helen had offered to drive us. When she came to pick us up I was surprised to learn that she had not felt the earthquake either.

As we drove along, I felt like my normal self, although I was still very euphoric which made the shopping trip especially fun. There seemed to be so many good deals to be had at the grocery store. I spent only sixty dollars, but from those purchases I was able to plan meals for the next two weeks. A speedy mind definitely seemed to be useful for grocery shopping and menu planning.

After driving home and unpacking the groceries we all sat down to lunch together. I then showed my cousin, Sabrina, around our apartment building. I had taken Sabrina outside, but when I attempted to punch in our room number so Mom could let us in, I found that it had completely slipped my memory. Some other tenants who were coming out of the building let us in, so there was nothing to worry about. But I couldn't believe it. How could I forget such a simple thing?

When Aunt Helen and Sabrina left for home, Mom and I spent the remainder of the day mostly just visiting. However, while Martina napped, we caught up on laundry, tidied the apartment, and prepared supper together. It was great having Mom's help cooking meals and keeping the apartment in order. It was sort of like old times, working together around the house.

Kurt arrived home from work that night in time for supper and we all enjoyed a leisurely meal, and then relaxed in front of the TV.

That night when Martina woke for her usual nighttime feeding, I nursed and changed her, then put her back to bed. I should have put myself back to bed too, but I again didn't feel tired. My mind was churning with creative ideas and I wanted to get them down on paper before I forgot them. Sitting at the kitchen table, I began to write fast and furiously. When I had finished, there was a great stack of papers on the table. There was a story for my nephew, songs I had made up to sing to Martina, and many poems. I had also made a list of books and topics from the Bible that I wanted to study. The majority of the writing was done in shorthand, which I hadn't used in about five years. My not sleeping did not concern me. I remember thinking that the apostle Paul probably didn't sleep much when he was writing in prison either. Maybe I didn't really need sleep. By then it was time for Kurt to get up for work so I made him his breakfast, all the while excitedly telling him about my writing.

Most of that next day, Wednesday, I spent at home, just talking with Mom. We talked about many different matters but the conversation would usually come back to my childhood; Mom was amazed at what I was suddenly remembering! My mind was recalling so much information and so many memories from my past, going back to when I was just a few years old. We apparently use only a small percentage of our brain—well, I seemed to be using much more of mine than usual.

The German language was also starting to come back to me. Although we had spoken German in my home when I was a very young child, before this time, what I had remembered was negligible. Now I was even able to sing "Silent Night" in German to Martina.

What I was experiencing at that time was mostly positive, at least emotionally, but I remember feeling an underlying anxiety. Some small part of me knew that what I was experiencing was not usual, and I wondered if I would ever feel "normal" again or if this feeling of building excitement would just continue. My mind was also beginning to feel tired and overcrowded from the thoughts and ideas that seemed to be moving faster and faster through it—like a runaway train about to crash. Even as a segment of my mind registered this feeling, the rest of me was carried along quite willingly.

Up to this point I was still perfectly able to care for Martina. In fact, I seemed especially sensitive to her needs. There was no question that we had bonded well. My relationship with Martina was all I could have hoped for. Like any mother, I changed, fed, bathed, and loved her. But there was a difference, a difference that I would feel more each day. Whereas a baby is usually the focal point in a new mother's life, I had no real focus. My mind was going in too many different directions. One minute I would be holding Martina and she would be the most precious and important thing in the world to me. The next minute, as my thoughts veered off in another direction, I would hardly be aware that she existed.

Later that afternoon Mom and I took Martina for a walk. We stopped in at the neighbourhood convenience store to pick up a few extra supplies for supper. Walking along, I felt a new confidence, a complete acceptance of who I was. There were no insecurities, no inhibitions; I felt perfect!

Supper that evening was a special affair. The table was

set with our fanciest dishes. I brought out candles and as a finishing touch placed a rose on the table, symbolizing our own special Martina Rose. I wanted the meal to be "just perfect," reflecting how I felt inside. It was so much fun using all of this previously dormant creativity. Normally I would not have had the energy or adrenalin to be constantly creating, constantly talking, and constantly doing, but I did at that time and I was enjoying it immensely.

All good things end some time: I didn't know it, but my euphoric balloon was about to pop. Although I had not been my typical self since coming home, there had really been nothing in my behaviour to make anyone feel that I was "sick." Prenatal classes had warned of possible "baby blues" but I was far from depressed! The events of that evening, however, made it apparent, especially to Kurt, that something was very wrong with me.

After supper, I drove Mom to a toy store in Richmond, leaving Martina sleeping at home with Kurt. I parked the car, and then realized that we were not at the correct location. Although we were still several blocks away, we decided to walk. At the store, I began impulsively buying gifts for my nephew and nieces, gifts which were not only unnecessary but which we could hardly afford at that time. I felt that with Martina getting so many gifts, they should have something special too so they wouldn't feel left out.

After purchasing the gifts, we proceeded to where I

thought the car was. It was not there. Suddenly I was completely disorientated. Whereas my mind had previously been so sharp and clear it now seemed to be lost in a fog. Where was the car? Where were we? It was a very frightening feeling. Mom had not paid close attention to where I had parked; she naturally assumed I knew where I was—but I didn't, not anymore. We walked back and forth, through back alleys, and down streets, but still no car.

In tears, I finally phoned Kurt from a phone booth. He in turn phoned Aunt Helen, who drove him and Martina to where we were. We got into my aunt's car. I felt not only very foolish but also afraid. I tried to picture where the car was—to think at all I needed to close my eyes—but each time we would drive to the location I mentioned, the car was not there. It was more like a bad dream than reality. We must have been driving around for well over an hour; patience was wearing thin all around and Martina was getting hungry. How Kurt ever managed it is beyond me, but eventually we did find the car.

It was a great relief to finally make it home that night but my strongest emotion was not relief but anger. I felt terribly angry. At who? Well, I guess at myself. Angry because my mind had been relaying so many crossed signals—angry, helpless, and afraid. I wanted to give an explanation for what had happened. I wanted there to be some reason, some excuse—but there was just no making sense of it. At home I sat in the rocking chair, nursing Martina, as the tears ran heedlessly down my cheeks.

After nursing Martina and getting her settled for the night, I took a bath and went off to bed myself, still trying to figure out how I could have possibly lost the car.

I felt somewhat better the next day, but my moods and behaviour were very unpredictable. I went from intense excitement over what the future might hold for me to a very real fear of what was happening to me. I talked incessantly to Mom all that day, then suddenly changed my behaviour completely when Kurt arrived home. I went into the bathroom and proceeded to throw everything from the counter into the bathtub. There was a loud clatter as brushes, makeup and bottles hit the tub. There was not any logical reason for doing what I did; I was not at all angry. Perhaps it was my way of making a not- so-silent plea for attention and help. It worked.

An appointment was made for me to see Dr. Davis at five o'clock. Since we had some time before the appointment, Kurt took me to the hairdresser for a much-needed haircut. It was a very enjoyable half-hour, at least for me. While my hair was being cut, I chatted away with the hairdresser, very openly and unself-consciously. She was soon telling me all about her life, family, and friends. As I looked in the mirror I could see Kurt in the waiting area, watching me intently. I'm sure he was wondering what on earth I might be saying to the hairdresser. Aside from buying some fifty dollars worth of conditioner, I did not act at all in a crazy way. I do remember thinking that it didn't really matter how much the conditioner cost. To my way of thinking, every time the phone rang, which was often in this hair salon, more money would appear in our checking account. I left feeling I had gotten a great deal.

When we got in to see Doctor Davis, Kurt told him about my behaviour since leaving the hospital. I also related to him some of what was happening from my point of view. He scribbled down notes as we talked, then left the office for a brief time, probably to look up my symptoms in his medical textbooks. On his return, Dr. Davis made an appointment for me at a health clinic for early the next morning. Because of my thyroid condition he felt it was important my thyroxin level be checked as severe hypothyroidism can cause psychosis. From that time on I was closely watched, either by Kurt, or Mom when he was at work. During the night when I would get up to feed Martina, Mom would be right there with me.

Friday morning at eight o'clock my blood tests were done. While at the medical office I behaved very sanely on the outside. I was able to answer all questions correctly and normally; however, what was going on internally was quite a different matter.

While the nurse took the blood sample from my arm I

paid close attention to exactly how she did it. I wanted to remember all the details for when I became a doctor. At one point I *heard* the nurse call me Doctor Ruhwald. When I was in the washroom giving a urine sample I was compelled to move the position of many items: a glass, paper towels, and soap—just a fraction. I was convinced I was a spy and that I needed to leave a message for the person who came in next because he/she might be a spy too.

The movements, especially the hand movements, of the people around me were special signals; even the signal lights and the honking of the cars outside had a special meaning.

I was obviously out of touch with reality at this time, yet the average person sitting in that office would not have known I was experiencing anything unusual at all. Mom certainly knew; I was sharing some of my *special insights* with her. I seemed to sense that it was *safe* to tell Mom what I was experiencing, while realizing that others would not accept it. When we arrived home following the appointment, Mom phoned Dr. Davis, explaining the events of the morning. His response was that I might possibly be going through what was called a "change of mind," which could happen with childbirth. The "change of mind" he referred to was just the opposite of postpartum depression. Dr Davis had already contacted a psychiatrist who was to call us sometime later that day.

The psychiatrist phoned that evening, suggesting: "Look, you can take Dorothy to emergency if necessary. Meanwhile, keep her off the thyroxin medication until the test results come in Tuesday."

Following the phone call, Kurt felt it would be best to take me to hospital right away. When he asked me my opinion, "Dorothy, do you want to go to the hospital? They can help you there,"

I responded, "Sure, there are lots of babies there!"

"This will be a different hospital than where you had Martina," Kurt tried to explain, "a hospital where the doctors will try to help you."

Help me? I didn't need help. But it would be nice to go among the patients and heal them, especially all the babies and children.

That I might need help or be sick was something I just couldn't understand. I knew everything around me was going crazy. What I was experiencing was very unusual, that was apparent even to me. But I had never had any reason to doubt my sanity before. Why should I start now? I just accepted my experience as reality—and it was very *real* to me.

In the end Kurt did not take me to hospital at that time. Mom persuaded him to wait a few days, since he had the weekend off and could help take care of me. It was very difficult for Mom to admit that I was so sick. She was, like any mother would, hoping and praying that I would get better without having to be admitted to the hospital's psychiatric ward.

I was not getting better though. In fact, daily I grew worse. It was like my rational mind was sinking into a quicksand of insanity. At first I had been able to flail about, temporarily catching on to a glimmer of reason and reality, but now I was well and truly sunk. Deep inside there was a part that was still the *real, normal* me, but to those who knew and loved me, I had completely vanished. The person they saw was not the Dorothy they knew. To them it was as if a stranger was living inside my body.

Now I needed constant supervision and care, both personally, such as in getting dressed, and in my maternal duties: feeding and caring for Martina. Friday night I did not sleep at all.

My memories of Saturday are very fragmented. I cannot write what happened in its proper sequence. I can only share with you, the reader, bits and pieces of what I was experiencing at that time.

Many of the ideas and thoughts I had were a conglomeration of what I had read recently, heard on the radio or watched on TV. Just weeks earlier, I had read a story which took place in Africa. As the sun was rising that Saturday morning, I laid on the couch in our living room looking out the window. I was really excited because, when the sun came up, I was sure we would find ourselves in Africa.

Often I would *hear* my father's voice, giving me advice on the silliest things such as how to clean the bathroom or make the bed properly. I found this very amusing, as Dad is not at all what anyone would call domestic. I would also sometimes *hear* Dad walk into the apartment and talk to Mom.

I remember hearing the voices of former teachers and pastors of mine. Sometimes there were so very many voices, all talking at once. This would have been enough to drive me crazy, if I had not already arrived.

At the time, one of the most interesting and enjoyable things for me to do was to watch TV. It came alive, with me as the main character. I remember watching a hockey game and feeling the excitement and exhilaration as *I* made the goal.

I didn't need the TV, though. There was enough *entertainment* going on inside my head. If I closed my eyes I could picture different shows in my head, from cartoons to nature films. One particularly vivid memory was of a baby deer in the woods. The beauty and detail of that picture, as I saw it, is impossible to describe completely. I could see the fawn as if it was truly right in front of me: it's twitching ears, big bright eyes; I could almost hear its heart beating. Then I saw a lion behind the deer. It gave a mighty roar—a roar that seemed to reverberate throughout my entire being.

Another time I had an image in my mind of a very young fetus inside the mother's womb, symbolizing to me the beginning of life. After that came pictures of people who had suffered in different ways: a woman who had been raped, a child who had been beaten, and a baby who had died from an abortion. I felt an intense pain inside, as if I had taken their pain upon myself. The sound of their screaming and crying filled my ears. The baby's cry, that of a newborn, stood out from the others, going on and on.

Religious delusions were also very prominent in my mind, a very common psychotic symptom. At times, I felt that it was the Second Coming, that Jesus Christ had come back in my body and was going to do wonderful things, including healing the sick and generally fixing all the problems in the world.

At other times I would be afraid that Kurt was possessed by Satan, or even that Satan might try to hurt Martina. I remember asking my mother to pray especially for protection for the baby. There was a great deal of fear involved in my illness at that time, fear for Kurt, Martina, and myself. The most frightening thing for me, however, was mind games, which I felt compelled to play. I needed to do specific and sometimes complicated things. For example: I needed to think of one hundred words starting with an A, then B, C..., on down through the alphabet, or I needed to find particles adding up to a large random number—these might be hairs on my head, rug fibres, or cells on my skin.

By playing these games I felt that somehow I was winning a fight against Satan. If I didn't play them, then Kurt or myself would die. On one occasion I was sitting on the couch and Kurt was sitting on the floor in front of me. I was frantically doing these games in my head while watching Kurt closely to make sure that he wasn't dying. At one point I felt that I needed to remain absolutely motionless. Then I felt that I really didn't need to play these games, that Satan just wanted to trick me. But always, I felt that if I made the wrong choice and lost "the game," I might die, resulting in the death of my family and eventually everyone on earth. These mental gymnastics were emotionally exhausting.

It was much like having the flu, being feverish and delirious during the night, when your dreams go around in circles. You wake up very tired. Well, I was certainly getting extremely tired, both physically and mentally, yet it was impossible for me to fall asleep. At one point Mom encouraged me to lie down and just rest, even if I couldn't sleep, but my eyes would not stay closed. I quickly got out of bed and opened the window wide. "If I jumped out," I thought," I bet I could fly away like a bird!" Fortunately, I didn't test my theory.

My illness had progressed beyond what Kurt or Mom could manage. It was not safe to have me remain at home any longer. That evening Kurt phoned the psychiatrist and made arrangements for me to be admitted to the hospital the next day.

Later that evening I talked to some members of my family on the phone. I was happy and excited to talk to them, but afterwards I became very quiet. Finally, on my own initiative, I went to bed and cried heartbrokenly, until completely exhausted, sleep finally came.

When Martina woke during the night for her feedings, she was given formula. Mom and Kurt wanted to give me a chance to get some much-needed sleep. I slept peacefully throughout the whole night, not waking until morning.

My bags were packed and I was ready to go. Just under a week after being released from hospital, I would be admitted again. However, this would be a different hospital, a different ward, and instead of a one-week stay, it would ultimately be my home for the next two and a half months. Ironically, it was Thanksgiving Weekend!

FOUR

The Ins and Outs of the Psychiatric Ward

*A*s we made the trip to hospital that Sunday morning, the car swirled with contrary emotions. I was filled with anticipation about where I might be going; Kurt and my mother definitely felt some trepidation. Although both Kurt and my mother's hearts were understandably heavy, I felt so light-hearted I seemed to be floating. There was classical music on the stereo; it filled my entire being till I felt ready to burst. As we went up and down the hills on the way to the hospital, I had the sensation of being on a musical roller-coaster ride.

Any thoughts I had regarding going to hospital were

very positive. I was going to help sick people. In fact, as we drove along I would blink at people and buildings, thinking I was somehow healing or blessing them.

When we arrived at the hospital I sat motionless, with my eyes shut. Kurt needed to lead me by the hand. While in the emergency room I *saw* people I had known as a child. Sitting on a chair between Kurt and my mother, I ever so slowly got up to walk away. Moving in slow motion, I felt sure no one would notice me leaving.

Finally, a nurse called my name and I was asked several questions to evaluate my condition. I was rational enough to give my complete address correctly. However, when asked why I was in hospital, my reply was: "They think I'm going crazy because I'm laughing so much."

After being assessed in emergency, I was then led to an examination room and left alone. I proceeded to take the room apart. If something could move, I moved it. If it could come off, well, it did. I was like an unsupervised toddler. Normally I would not have dreamt of touching anything, but I was far from my normal self. My inhibitions, which protected me and guided my behaviour, were gone.

When Mom came in so I could nurse Martina, she found me sitting on the bed in a hospital gown, my clothing all tucked underneath. I took no initiative in feeding the baby; Mom had to hold Martina to my breast so she could nurse.

After nursing Martina, I was taken to the Psychiatric Ward for further assessment. The three of us met with a psychiatric team consisting of a psychiatrist, psychiatric nurses, and a social worker. We all sat in a circle and were given a chance to share our thoughts and feelings on the situation. As the psychiatrist asked me questions I watched her closely. She was a professional looking black woman with bright red nail polish. Although she was very kind, I felt unable to trust her. I could *see* blood running out of her fingertips down the arms of the chair. Every once in a while she would look down and begin busily writing:

> *Department of Psychiatry, Progress Record:*
>
> *Admitted via wheelchair 23-year-old Caucasian, married woman, nearly 2 weeks post delivery of first child. Dorothy was only minimally responsive during admission to the ward. Mood changeable. Inappropriate answers and bizarre behaviors noted. Not oriented to date, time or place. No valuables or sharps. Placed on CONSTANT OBSERVATION.*

Following the assessment I was taken by wheelchair to my room in psychiatric ward B. This too was an exciting ride. We seemed to be racing, faster and faster, around corners, up stairs. I felt the need to hang onto the arms of my chair, lest I go flying out.

When I was settled in my room, a doctor came in to give me a physical. Kurt and Mom went to the cafeteria for lunch. Upon returning to the nursing station, they were informed that I would be put on medication -Haloperidol- because of my behaviour. Entering my room to say goodbye, they found me sitting on an unmade bed. The sheets and the plastic padding from the headboard had been torn off. Wrapped in the sheets was my lunch tray along with all my plastic utensils.

My mother took me into her arms, crying, "Dorothy, they're trying to help you... goodbye, Dorothy."

The doctor tried to reassure her, "It's OK, she's doing her very best."

Mom walked out, crying. As the tears came, she struggled to believe that God was still in control, that with so many people praying this must somehow be within His will.

Kurt had Martina admitted into the hospital's nursery for the night, until more permanent arrangements could be made. Then they both left for home. Kurt had mixed feelings about leaving me in hospital, but at that time it was largely relief. It had been a tremendous burden and responsibility to watch over me twenty-four hours a day, wondering what I would do next. Finally I was where I could get help.

Patient resistive to writer's attempts to move her to another room, closer to nursing station. Kicking and striking out at staff but eventually settled enough to be escorted to new room. Once in bed began making constant motions with her hands. Responded only once to staff—when asked what baby's name was.

Carl, a male nurse, was sitting in a chair flipping through a magazine while keeping a watchful eye on me sitting in bed. From my point of view I was in a bizarre sort of prison and Carl was my prison guard. He represented Satan and to make him go away I needed to do specific things such as move my feet or clap my hands. I could clearly see the unease in his eyes. It would be hard to say who was more afraid at that time, him or I.

Part of what made me suspicious of these so—called nurses was there difference to any nurses I had seen before. They wore no uniforms, just casual clothing. Male nurses were also unfamiliar to me and the psychiatric ward had several. Some of the nurses seemed really evil; I thought of them as black, others were grey—fighting between their good and bad sides.

In this foreign environment, I didn't feel able to trust anyone. Sure, I was psychotic and a lot of what was going on inside my head made me feel as though I was involved in a bizarre game. But deep inside there was the *real me*, feeling terribly hurt, lonely, afraid, and angry. I had lost my husband, my baby, and my possessions—everything that gave me a sense of my identity—and been put in a foreign environment where I felt incapable of doing what was expected of me. I was in some sort of a jail yet what crime had I committed.

> *Very tearful and upset... calling out and crying occasionally throughout the evening. Very resistive to oral meds. Hallucinating. Given reassurance that her child was safe in the nursery here; she does not appear to believe this.*

I found the medication very difficult to swallow. I also didn't know what they might me giving me. In my mind it could be poison. Sometimes I would spit it out onto my gown or into my hand and hope the nurses wouldn't notice.

That evening my thyroxin and pituitary hormone levels were taken, to explore a possible hormonal cause to the psychosis. However, even at that time, the endocrinologist, Dr. Tyler, did not think it was an endocrine problem.

I remember lying completely covered underneath my hospital blanket. Looking through the fibres, I could see people, more than likely nurses, moving around. To me, it all seemed like a puppet show.

The next day, Monday, Mom flew home. When Kurt came to visit me, I still didn't have a clue why I was in hospital.

> *Patient agitated and weeping several times, appeared to be answering auditory hallucinations, very groggy following medication.*
>
> *Husband visited. Appeared very supportive and concerned. She recognized him and answered somewhat appropriately for a short time then grew angry and swore at him.*

When Kurt would come to visit me in the evenings I would often be very upset. There was really nothing he could do except try to reassure and comfort me, and he did, but it was futile. No amount of encouragement could get through to me. He felt helpless and frustrated. My pastor also stopped by for a while, but I didn't respond to him in any way. I simply sat quietly and stared straight ahead.

On Tuesday I was transferred to psychiatric ward A. There was still a nurse sitting with me constantly, either in my room or in the recreation room if I was watching TV.

An endocrinologist came in the next day. My blood test results showed my thyroxin level was normal; I apparently no longer needed the thyroxin medication I had been taking for several years. This was very significant since after a radioactive iodine treatment when I was 18 for *hyper*thyroidism I had become *hypo*thyroid. In other words, my thy-roxin level was low so I needed to supplement it with thy-roid hormones. Although the cause of my psychosis was not an endocrine problem, my body had quite obviously changed the amount of hormones my thyroid gland was putting out.

Patient was struggling with her sitter, Appar-ently she had kicked him a few times and had wanted to leave the unit. Given firm redirec-tion. Placed in restraints due to further acting out.

Being put into restraints during the next few days was a very common occurrence, although it is just a very dim memory. I do, however, remember fighting to leave and being afraid the nurses were injecting me with poison. Normally, I am anything but a violent person, but during the first days in hospital, my behaviour was at times quite violent and out of control. To me I was fighting for my life. Questions running through my crazed mind were: Where am I? Where is my baby? I would often become quite agi-tated about Martina, wondering where she was.

Left wrist noted to be very bruised around area where the restraint was. Hips also red-dened and bruised in areas of I.M.

Had to be placed back in wrist restraints due to lack of control... when staff attempted to get her contact lenses from her, she squirted staff with the solutions.

At this time I was still unwisely wearing my contacts. Having no concept of time, I would often leave them in for long periods of time, even sleeping with them in my eyes. After many attempts made by the hospital staff, I finally took them out.

Accepted meds with no resistance although spat out lunch meds due to foul taste. Has been fascinated with baths (has taken 3)

Other patients would often ask, " So, Dorothy...how many baths have you had today?" then laugh when I told them the number. I would take several baths during the day. Even during the night when other patients were peacefully sleeping, I would bang on the locked door to the bath area, trying to get in.

Remains vague, illogical. Understands she is in hospital due to her behaviour but is unable to identify which behaviours caused her to be put into hospital.

Eventually, it got through to me that I was not in hospital to help others but I still didn't realize I was sick or needed help. The nurses would often ask me questions, sort of like a reality check, to try to make me understand, but it just wouldn't sink in.

My Mom and Dad made the trip to Vancouver to visit me, arriving the next Saturday. By then I had been in hospital 6 days. They first visited Martina at our apartment in Richmond, where Kurt's mother was now looking after her. When Dad first saw me he was shocked; he hadn't thought it would be *that* bad. Mom had explained what I had been experiencing but nothing could truly prepare him for what he saw. Although I recognized them, I seemed quite indifferent towards both him and Mom. I was obviously very drugged, in a daze, with my eyelids half closed.

"You'll get well soon and go home with your baby," my father choked out; "…you've got a very nice baby."

"Oh, I've got lots more babies," I blithely replied.

I went through Mom's purse, took out her bankbook and added quickly, but completely inaccurately. "You've got a million dollars in your account," I stated proudly, as if I had caused the money to miraculously appear. I then abruptly stood up and left the room.

Dorothy in with her parents holding a pink baby blanket rocking it as though she had her baby in her arms. Stated "I'm doing so much better now that I have my baby." Parents both appeared quite stressed sitting quietly with Dorothy.

Since my parents had come to hospital, I felt sure they would take me home. I packed up my belongings, left my room, and sat on a chair, waiting for them to take me away.

Dorothy found sitting outside of the elevator on the 5th. floor. Dorothy stated when asked where she had gone "to hell." Dorothy was put into restraints and settled.

When Kurt visited me that weekend and found out about my leaving the ward he was understandably concerned. The staff tried to reassure him about watching me closely, but realistically, they couldn't watch me every single second. On all of the tranquilizers I was on, most people would not be able to move, let alone try to run away. But these drugs did not seem to slow me down as far as leaving the ward went. A doctor later told me that the amount of drugs I was on would have stopped a full grown elephant in its tracks. He may have been exaggerating but the point was clear. Later, a nurse jokingly told me that I had been a real slippery character. In a way that made me feel proud that I had the gumption to try and escape, since I am naturally quite shy and intimidated in new surroundings.

*Baby in—Dorothy showed appropriate con-
cern and caring however she wanted to breast
feed the child and would not accept medical
reasons forbidding her to do so (was however
dissuaded).*

*Trust remains a problem. She does follow
direction from her husband.*

*Did spend some time with other female
patients and appeared to enjoy this.*

When my parents came in to visit on Monday they noticed that I seemed a bit better, more alert, and not nearly as
drugged.

*Improvement noted. AWOL risk reduced—
has made no attempts to leave. Able to con-
verse appropriately for very brief periods
however still is grossly disorganized. Facial
affect somewhat more animated, appears to
be more aware of her environment. Still no
insight.*

That evening I visited several hours with Kurt, and before he left I asked him if I could leave and go home. By the
next day I was able to go to the washroom and back with no
supervision and my conversation was more integrated but
only for brief periods of time.

*AWOL to _____ St., returned to unit by se-
curity.*

So much for my big improvement! When my parents
visited me that day, they found me going through other patients' belongings and wearing their clothes.

In my eyes, these clothes belonged to me. I was again
like a toddler and everything centered on me—everything
was mine!

> *Wed. Oct. 21—Transferred to Ward B ac-
> companied by staff, co-operative to the trans-
> fer. Patient has no insight, states "They (the
> devils + angels) brought me here." Told writer
> that she has twins, a boy and a girl, ... is dis-
> oriented and delusional. Conversation vague
> and appears preoccupied although denies ex-
> periencing visual and auditory hallucina-
> tions.*

I was in a hospital gown but I would often try my own
clothes on, which were stored in a duffel bag. I ended up
losing some of my clothes in the move to psychiatric ward
B, as well as other clothing in the laundry room.

The nurses rightly wanted patients to be responsible for
their own possessions but it was not possible in my case.
What really frustrated Kurt was the hospital staff not dis-

tinguishing between what I was capable of and what other patients could do. Someone with an eating disorder can obviously look after their own clothing and possessions; however, you just couldn't rightly expect a 2 year old to be that responsible, let along someone in the midst of a psychosis.

When the nurses finally became aware that I was losing my clothing it was put into my locker and locked up. I remember being extremely frustrated, trying over and over again to get into the locker.

Has difficulty comprehending simple instructions, constantly asking for her clothes and not able to remember her room number. Presents an AWOL risk. Remains in P.J.'s and close observation. Found wandering into other patient's room.

I found it very disorientating to be often changing rooms and wards. Once I left my bedroom there was no guarantee I could find my way back. Having my parents visit was also in a sense confusing to me. I was in a very strange environment, yet my parents, seemingly from a completely different world, kept appearing, and then leaving again. I couldn't understand what part they played in this strange drama. Were they going to help me escape or not?

Thurs. Oct. 22—Appears to be hallucinating visually and experiencing delusions. Was adamant that a stuffed moose (miniature) in the patients' lounge was "waving his ears." She said as she coughed in this writer's presence: I have to cough low because if the moose hears me he'll think it's a mating call." Laughed copiously. Pale in coloring. Needing close supervision, as she tended to wander and pick up objects from the desk....

...was decided to restrict visitor to husband only. Medication changed to Mellaril to stabilize mental status.

When my parents came in to visit me that day they were told it would be better for me if they didn't come back, to just say goodbye briefly. Before they left for home, they stopped in to see me for a few minutes, dropping off some cookies and writing materials. Following their visit I was slightly agitated but the nursing staff was able to settle me down with reassurance.

By the weekend I still showed no real positive affect from the change in medication to Mellaril. It had been two long weeks and I was still trapped in a state of psychosis. The small *real me* inside felt that if I could just escape the hospital and find my way back home to Kurt, my life would change back to normal. Of course in my condition I never would have found my way home.

I did make it outside the hospital building, at least twice. One particular time is very clear to me. I remember opening a door and running downstairs, hearing a loud clacking sound echoing in my head as my slippers hit each step. My heart was beating wildly as I opened the outside door and ran onto the hospital lawn. I didn't get far, thankfully. Downtown Vancouver is not the safest place for anyone, let alone a crazy lady dressed in nothing but a hospital gown. I was caught by several nurses and dragged kicking and swearing back into the hospital where I was tranquilized and restrained. I was incredibly angry and afraid. To me I was fighting for my life.

I realized my parents couldn't take me home and I couldn't pull off an escape myself, but perhaps Kurt could somehow sneak me out of hospital. One evening when he came to visit I thought he was going to do just that. On this occasion I had taken a pop, which belonged to another patient, from the fridge in the patient's kitchen. When Kurt came to visit me that evening he asked permission to take me to the cafeteria. The staff agreed, so off we went.

In my state of mind I was sure Kurt had very cunningly figured out the perfect plan to get me out of hospital. He had told me we were just going to the cafeteria but I felt certain we were finally making the big escape. To Kurt I was acting silly, prancing down the hallway with a silly grin on my face, but what I felt inside was quite different.

My heart was beating hard as we walked down the hallway. I felt excited, but also afraid and anxious. "Would we really be able to get away with this?"

When we arrived at the cafeteria, Kurt bought the pop. To my complete disbelief and horror we headed right back towards the Psychiatric Ward. I could *hear* the doctor's and nurse's voices as they walked by us. The dialogue went something like this:

"I don't believe it! He's taking her back!" "Why doesn't he get her out of here?!" "This is his big chance!.".. *"Well, that's it. He'll never get her out now."*

Back in my room again I felt sick, as if there was a big rock resting in the pit of my stomach. I also felt angry, frustrated and defeated. All of these emotions were released in a flood of tears. Kurt's primary emotion at that time was probably surprise. I had not confided a word to him about what he was *supposedly* planning. He showed a lot of compassion towards me at that time but somehow it was just not enough. I felt he was now powerless to help me get out of hospital. This bothered me, as he had always seemed to be in control. He had always been looking after me. Now the nurses were in control and he was unable to help me escape from this nightmarish situation.

FIVE

Expectations

*A*fter trying unsuccessfully to escape, and realizing that Kurt could not break me out of hospital, I possibly resigned myself to staying. For the most part I made no further attempts to leave.

> *Oct. 27—Close Observation Continues.*
> *Thought disorder only apparent in prolonged conversation—able to carry on appropriate superficial conversations—more involved with self-care. Some sense of humor evident. Looking forward to visit with husband.*

When I was expecting a visit from Kurt, I would try to make myself look as nice as possible. This was quite difficult as my wardrobe consisted of hospital gowns. I did, however, like the yellow ones; they were rather pretty. I once wore a flower in my hair. Who knows whom I *borrowed* it from?

Some of the other female patients would sometimes do my hair, or even apply my makeup. On occasion I would go into the room set aside for patients to do their hair and makeup. I would sit there for what seemed like hours, fully expecting someone to just miraculously show up and give me a makeover. Once I got bored with waiting in the chair and made an intricate roadway all over the room with curlers.

"Did you do this?" asked a patient in amusement upon entering the room.

"Yes!" I stated with great pride. In my eyes it was a wonderful accomplishment full of symbolism and hidden meaning.

Oct 28—Up wandering along hallway at 0330 hrs. States she heard the baby crying.

Behaviour restless as not able to sit still for more than approx. 2 min. However, did remain in "thought stopping" and "self esteem" meetings.

Life in the psychiatric ward during the weekdays was very structured. In the mornings there were community meetings to attend. All the patients and as many of the staff as possible would attend these meetings. The purpose of these meetings was for everyone to air concerns, discuss program plans and make decisions regarding the operation of the ward. While I was psychotic I had great difficulty with these meetings. For one thing I found it next to impossible to find my way to the meeting place, which was downstairs, unless another patient or staff member took me at the correct time.

If I had been absolutely sane I would still have had a hard time, the two major reasons being I was not wearing a watch or my contact lenses. My vision was very poor, so poor that I couldn't even tell time on the large clocks in the hallway of the hospital. I remember trying to tell time on my hospital wristband. Other patients got quite a kick out of it. Once they asked me what time it was. I was surprisingly close and they all laughed hilariously.

If I did find my way, alone, to the room where the meeting was being held, it was invariably late, which of course didn't meet with the approval of the rest of the *community*. With my psychosis I also had absolutely no concept of time. Morning, afternoon, day, or night; it made no difference to me. I just had no idea. And yet I was expected to take the responsibility of getting myself to these meetings on time, being watchless, sightless, and practically witless! Although outwardly I was simply responding to the psychosis, the *real me* deep inside found this very frustrating and stressful, being expected to do what I felt incapable of doing.

I remember on one occasion being in the basement where there was a large kitchen, an eating room, and different meeting and activity rooms. I had probably been told that it was time for a meeting but I couldn't find the right room. I was very afraid, walking from room to room, hearing strange noises. Whether or not I found the right room that time I don't know but more than likely I eventually did, late again.

At the community meetings everyone present would be seated in a circle of chairs. To start with, everyone would say his or her name. I wasn't sure if this was a game of some kind or what. What kind of answer were they expecting from me? I just picked one of the names I heard mentioned, and repeated it. With much prompting from the leader, I realized they wanted *my* name. But which one should I give them? I decided on Dorothy Schlitt, my maiden name. Also, I thought this game might possibly be like musical chairs; I would often get up during the meeting and move to an empty chair. It was very difficult for me to endure an entire meeting. Not only was I restless and unable to concentrate on what was going on around me, but I often felt extremely hot and dizzy with buzzing in my ears, possibly a side affect of the medication. I remember just staring at the pattern in the carpet hoping the meeting would quickly end.

Different patients each day would have the opportunity to be chairperson and secretary of these community meetings. Once I was asked to be secretary, which made me feel quite proud. Needless to say, in my psychotic state, the minutes that day were very unusual, even including an acrostic poem. Later, after I came out of the psychosis, I got a chance to read them. Although I laughed at the time, inside I felt just sick; it was a look at insanity I wished to forget.

Mealtime was another part of the hospital schedule I had difficulty with. The first while I had a tremendous appetite. I would ask Kurt to bring me milkshakes, chocolate bars, and hamburgers. The hospital food tasted terribly bland and I found it almost impossible to swallow their oatmeal cookies. They were so very dry. I felt sure they were trying to choke me to death.

Meals seemed to come at random times. For quite a while I took meals by myself upstairs in the patients' kitchen instead of downstairs with the others. I would sometimes hunt around for my food, and see a tray with half eaten food on it. Was this my meal? I thought they were trying to play a trick on me. Finally I would be shown to where I was to eat and be given my food. I could be shown where to go every day, but there would be no guarantee that I would remember. Sometimes I thought the nurses were trying to poison me with the food they gave me. There were strange round shiny things in the juice (ice from still being a bit frozen).

My condition was obviously not completely understood and my abilities differentiated from the other patients. Several patients had eating disorders, or were depressed; they still had all or most of their mental faculties available. Naturally, they could be held more accountable than myself and other psychotic patients. Although the nurses had difficulty knowing my limits (after all, they hadn't known me before I was sick), Kurt had no trouble realizing that I was incapable of responsibility. In his eyes I was a completely different person. Dorothy was gone.

Oct. 29—Husband in to visit. He talked with staff re: his worries—How

> *long will it take for his wife to get better? Her "values" and "thoughts" expressed now are so different from how she used to be. He's worried that her values are changing.— Reassured that these thoughts are all part of her illness and that as she gets better they will leave.*

> *Dorothy escalated when Kurt appeared—*

pacing about—looking for her baby in others'
rooms.

Aside from daily community meetings, on different days throughout the week there were also goal setting groups, therapy groups, self-run groups, task groups, elective groups, and recreation groups. Yes, quite a full schedule. I didn't attend all of these groups while I was psychotic but one in particular I remember very clearly. A small group of patients, myself included, were asked to make a drawing. There was music playing in the background. I'm not normally artistic but the music seemed to inspire me. I have never enjoyed drawing so much. My pencil didn't stop moving from the time the music started to when it stopped. My picture turned out to be very elaborate with the crucifixion scene of Christ symbolized.

Oct 30, mental status interview: Dorothy was
able to tolerate approx. 45 mins without
wanting to leave or be agitated... alert and re-
sponsive, knows name and place, does not
know date. Dorothy states: "thoughts in my
head are too many and it's difficult for me to
know what to respond to." Flight of ideas also
evident in conversation, preoccupied with
thoughts of religious content: black/white
sides, good/ bad and thoughts of where baby

is. Spoke about having two children... Delu-
sional thinking evident, as she believes she
has telepathic abilities and she "makes" all
people. Evidence of week ego boundaries—
confusion about who is her husband and who
is herself. Lacks insight as states " I'm in hos-
pital to help other people." Mood—
changeable, swings from smiling to almost
crying.

In my spare time I was usually watching TV or sitting in the patients' lounge listening to music on the radio. Music when I was psychotic was absolutely incredible. Although outwardly I would sit very quietly with maybe a toe or two wiggling in time to the music, inwardly it was all encompassing. I breathed in time with the music, just *knowing* that it was myself keeping the music going. I felt that I had written, sung, and produced all music on the radio.

One evening there was a concert being held for patients in hospital. I was expecting a friend to visit that evening so decided to go just for a while. A man was playing an accordion; again; I was very involved with the music. I was sure my mind was controlling his hands, playing the music. Ironically, when I got up to leave he stopped playing. I thought, "See, that proves it; I am controlling the music!"

When I wasn't listening to music in the patients' lounge

I would often visit with other patients or leaf through magazines, circling or making check marks on everything that I desired—mostly clothes. My plan was to purchase the marked items when I left hospital. I felt sure the nurses had piles of my 'new' clothes behind the locked door where they kept the medication.

I would sometimes also sit in my room and write at great length: poems, acrostics, anything that came to mind. They didn't make a bit of sense to me after I came out of the psychosis. At the time, however, my writing seemed to be very important gems of enlightenment and knowledge.

At one time I asked Kurt to bring me my Bible. He brought me an older one of his and I did some reading in the Song of Solomon. I had some very interesting but un-biblical interpretations of scripture. I would take my Bible to the patients' lounge and discuss my *ideas* with another patient, who also attended church.

Because I didn't have a very long attention span I would often walk from the patients' lounge to the TV room, then back again, over and over. I distinctly remember one night feeling as if I was walking right through the walls.

Other patients were able to at least leave the hospital for brief periods on a supervised walk each afternoon. Because of my escape attempts, I was naturally not one of them. I would watch longingly as the other patients went out each afternoon. I felt sure they were managing to escape but they always came back.

> *Nov. 2—More subdued today. Cooperative in following ward routines. Dorothy is more appropriate generally and can carry on a conversation for longer period without getting into delusional material.*
>
> *Visited by husband and baby this afternoon. Dorothy appears still unsure of herself but is showing motivation and interest in dealing with the baby.*

One nurse found out that I knew how to knit, so she gave me some knitting needles and helped me knit a baby bonnet. Although I had knit a baby blanket during my pregnancy with Martina, it was as if I had to learn all over again. My mind was very sluggish; casting on the yarn was impossible. The nurse was very patient, spending a lot of time helping me, all the while talking about how Martina could wear this little bonnet. But I just couldn't accept and grasp the reality of Martina wearing the bonnet. After all, my mind was as tangled and knotted as my knitting project. There would need to be a lot of straightening out in the threads of my mind before life could come together again in any semblance of normalcy.

Nov. 4—Superficially friendly and conversation more appropriate, especially while working on knitting project.

Some inappropriate behaviour this afternoon—observed folding bath towels + placing several of these in her bed. Also stated "Someone keeps grabbing my foot." ...seen taking things from the lounge (plants, juices and paper towels) and hoarding them in her room....tried to spit out her meds. Needs to be on liquid meds.

I often had a lot of difficulty sleeping at night. Because I had no concept of time I would wander around, going into the bathrooms to try and take a bath. Or I would make my way into the kitchen for a midnight snack: sandwiches and coffee (which normally I can't stand).

Getting up during the night and raiding the kitchen was generally frowned upon but I guess there wasn't much the staff could do, aside from forcibly making me go back to bed. One night on my trip to the kitchen the nurse called out from his station: "Dorothy, you're supposed to be in bed!"

"I'm hungry!" I replied, and then proceeded to make my sandwich.

"Dorothy... shut the lights off." Was this supposed to

deter me? Obediently I shut the kitchen lights off, continuing with my sandwich building by the light coming from the open fridge.

Back in my room I would look out the window, feeling very bored, waiting for the lights in the surrounding buildings to come back on. I would lie down for a while, then sit at the window, listening until I'd hear sounds of the construction workers outside. I felt that I was what started the construction each morning, like an unseen foreman. On one occasion I wrote notes and threw them out of my window, which only opened a crack. I hoped someone would read my message and help me. I can just imagine some construction worker finding one of these pieces of paper, reading it, looking up at the windows, shaking his head, and saying, "Yup, that's the Psych. ward alright."

SIX

No End in Sight

For the most part delusional thinking so overpowered my mind that thoughts of Martina were pushed out. However, even in the midst of psychosis, my maternal instinct found an outlet. I felt that all the babies and children on television were mine.

> *Nov. 5—Remains on close observation. Appears more sedated and aggressive as compared to last week. Delusional thinking continues: talking of twins, 2 babies and someone must have murdered one of them. Spends free time writing "delusional" notes. Attended and stayed for activity in afternoon. Taking*

notice in her appearance as she applied make-up.

When Martina did come in for a visit I found it difficult to believe that this was the same baby I had given birth to. She didn't look at all the same. Martina was now bigger, chubbier, and had a bit of a rash on her face. I also couldn't understand why she was so bundled up. Martina was wrapped in blankets, wore a hat, and two sleepers. I was afraid she might be suffocating with all those clothes. Of course I didn't realize that it was colder outside, now being November, than when I had been admitted, when it was still like summer. Perhaps I had twins, a boy and a girl. This must be a boy since it looked so different from my new-born. Kurt had the baby bundled up so I couldn't tell that this was the boy. So my line of logic went.

Kurt assured me that there was just one baby, Martina, and encouraged me to unwrap her and see for myself, that yes, this was my little girl.

Nov. 6—Dorothy appeared to lose her balance and fell to her knees. B.P. taken—84/60. Denied feeling light headed. ...sleepy and aggressive...fell asleep sitting up in task meeting...refused to attend community meeting or to take on a task.

Kurt came to visit me almost every night, when he wasn't flying out of town. There came a time, however, when he realized that for his own emotional health, he needed to take some time alone, away from the whole situation. He went to a cousin's cabin a couple of weekends, just relaxing, hiking, even chopping wood. Anything to relieve the intense stress he had been under. Kurt, like most husbands, is a fixer. But my illness was not something he could fix. He needed to just let go, and trust the hospital staff to do their best for me. His part was to support me as best he could. And that was something he definitely did.

Kurt was always very accepting of me when he came to visit. In the whole time I stayed at hospital I can only remember one other spouse of a patient coming to visit them and those visits were few and far between. It would have been very easy for Kurt to just leave me at the hospital with the attitude "Well, I'll see you if and when you come through this," but he didn't. He stuck with me the whole way.

I always looked forward to Kurt's visits, especially when he brought Martina in. On my birthday, November 6, Kurt brought her to visit all dressed up in a pretty pink dress, with matching knitted jacket, bonnet, and booties. To celebrate he brought a carrot cake with cream cheese icing which he had made himself, and balloons. The cake was passed out among the other patients and staff. I would never have known it was my birthday if Kurt hadn't told me but he took the effort to make it very special for me. He showed me that I was still his wife, and still an important person in his life.

Dorothy appeared settled following visit of husband and baby. Denied that today was her birthday. Wandering about unit holding balloons.

In my psychotic state Martina was still important to me, especially at certain times, but generally she was in the background. My memories of the visits with her are merely like snapshots. I remember showing Martina to the nurses. A grandmotherly patient came into my room once when Martina was there. Having a baby, something brand new and so vitally alive, in such a place, was so special to her. Although I allowed her to briefly hold Martina, I remember being afraid she might drop her.

Nov. 7—Mental status unchanged. Refused her meds, insistent that staff take it "if it's so good." Continued to refuse despite encouragement and was resistive to an injection. Appeared very paranoid. Finally received injection of Haldol 20 mg with four staff present.

I'm sure I also missed Kurt a lot when he was unable to visit. Possibly for this reason I felt that all of the male nurses had facets of Kurt's personality in them. It was a way for me to always feel his presence. So I enjoyed Kurt's visits, but even when he wasn't there, to me he still was, in a sense, only in different people.

> *Nov. 8—Husband stated his intention to phone ward tomorrow regarding his concerns about Dorothy not receiving thyroid replacement medication. He is expressing anxiety at Dorothy's lack of progress...*

I also saw different members of my family in other patients. The grandmotherly patient who was so interested in Martina reminded me so much of Kurt's mother. I spent many hours visiting with her. There were also two male patients who I felt were my older brothers, Wilfred and Peter. Possibly seeing members of my family in others made me feel a little less alone.

I remember on one occasion we had a new female patient come in. To me, it was Wilfred in disguise. I found it incredibly funny that my brother would sneak in hospital to visit me disguised as a female patient, wearing a skirt no less. He had gained a lot of weight in certain areas but their personalities were strikingly similar.

Nov. 9—Husband visited this evening and says he spoke with Dr. G___ earlier. Seems more reassured. Visit with husband and baby went well. Less inappropriate behaviour noted—seems pre-occupied at times— pleasant when approached. Conversation appropriate on superficial level. Remains on close observation.

I would quite often phone members of my family long distance. Our topics of conversation were, if completely off the wall, at least interesting and often humorous. I talked to Wilfred of having Bible Studies with the apostles, and that Paul had a great sense of humor. I spoke with my brother Peter in great detail and with conviction of Sylvester Stallone and Jesus Christ visiting me in hospital. Jesus had shown me the nail wounds in His hands; they had healed very well. I was proud that not only a modern celebrity, but Jesus Christ himself had taken the time to visit me.

Although our conversations were crazy, at least my end of them, family members were always willing to take my calls. Knowing it was their daughter/sister who was so nuts, I'm sure, made them feel just sick inside. But they never showed their natural aversion and fear of my illness by rejecting me.

Nov 10—Dorothy remains flagrantly psychotic in her thinking...observed to be laughing to herself, appears to be responding to hallucinations.

Blood work for thyroid abnormal, thyroid replacement has now been ordered.

I also received calls from family as well. They were in a sense a lifeline I could hold onto, keeping me in touch with 'normal' people in the real world who were still the same and cared about me as before. My mind the first while in the hospital was quite sharp; I had several phone numbers memorized. As the psychosis progressed, however, I found it impossible to figure out how to even use the phone.

Nov. 11—More disorganized today, actively psychotic, inappropriate in affect, moved to new room to be closer to nursing station, agitated at times, has taken at least 4 baths today, appears also to be more disoriented to ward. Speak with Dr. Is she toxic? Little social interaction. States she is "worried about baby" and is uncertain as to who is looking after her. States she is aware that there are periods when her "mind goes blank and I don't remember things."

I found it easier to process my phone conversations with family into my life in hospital, than my visits with Martina. It was a great treat for me to see her but it was also disconcerting. I felt that perhaps the nurses were teasing me with her. Martina would be with me for a short while, then gone. This could be a way for the nurses to get to me. I really didn't know quite how to react.

I did want Martina with me but part of me was afraid to even touch her, let alone hold or feed her. That part of me, the 'real' Dorothy, was afraid to give myself to her emotionally. It was easier to just keep a safe distance and not feel anything at all. I can still remember Martina lying on my bed. She looked up at me with her great big round eyes and smiled. Here was my beautiful baby, obviously happy and satisfied. And she didn't need me. She had reality—safe, normal life with Dad and Oma. And here I was living in a nightmare. I would have liked so much to step over the line into reality and go home with Kurt, and be a mother to my baby, but I couldn't. Each time as Kurt left with Martina, I remained, alone.

Nov. 17—Dr. G ___: probable Bipolar Affective Disorder (Manic) precipitated by childbirth. Will add lithium carbonate. Interview with Kurt—note: during the interview Dorothy appeared embarrassed by the discussion *of her behavior. There is considerable warmth and love between the two of them. Kurt is very concerned about her welfare, but reasonably so. Dorothy can be held to the topic and be rational for several sentences at a time, then admits her mind "gives in."*

When Kurt learned that the Dr. had decided to treat me with lithium he was pleased. He had done research at the library, looking through medical textbooks to find out anything he could on postpartum psychosis. Although there was a pitifully small amount of information available, Kurt had noted the case of a mother who had postpartum psychosis where lithium treatment had worked very well. So after six weeks of a psychosis, the change in medical treatment gave him new hope.

SEVEN

Waking Up

Nov. 19—Lithium therapy started this a.m. No significant change in mental status since Haldol discontinued this a.m. Appears drowsy and tired at times. Spending time in lounge with co-patients, attending groups, remains on close observation.

*A*ny positive results from the lithium were definitely not instantaneous. In fact two days after the start of lithium Kurt was very concerned that I was getting worse. When he came to visit me I became very angry with him, demanding that he take me home. The third day after the start of lithium treatment, however, things began to click. In a period of one day I went from being completely out of touch with reality to sanity, something I hadn't felt for awhile.

Nov. 22—0730-1930: Drowsy, subdued most of shift. Limited social interaction with co-patients noted. States she is in hospital "to help other patients." When reminded that she is in the patient role here, Dorothy quickly responded "something went wrong with my mind following delivery. It may have something to do with the amount of blood I lost." Recalls being very "confused and hyper" prior to admission. Appeared tearful during 1:1 today.

1930-2400: Dorothy's mental status is significantly clearer tonight, no evidence of delusional thinking. Her affect is remarkably brighter and appropriate, more easily engaged in conversation, she subjectively reports feeling better "I'm not blaming anyone" "I'm starting to feel more like myself." "Know I only have one baby" Interacting more with co-patients actually asked co-patients to lead in a singsong.

To me it was as if a fog was slowly being lifted from my

mind or as if I was slowly waking up from a bad dream. Just as when you sleep too long, you feel groggy upon awakening, in the same way I was basically awake (sane) that day yet it took several days for me to completely understand reality. Just as bad dreams often stay with you several hours after awakening, it took me a while to really understand that what I had been experiencing was not in fact reality.

When Kurt visited me that evening he asked me several questions to see if I was really out of the psychosis or was still suffering from delusional thinking. Although I did now realize that I was in the psychiatric ward of a hospital, I had no true understanding of what had actually happened to cause me to be there. Kurt explained that I had suffered postpartum psychosis but this was difficult for my mind to digest. I felt that I might still be in control of the music on the radio and the shows on TV. My delusions had been so strong; my brain had held them as truth for so long, that even though logically I knew they were purely delusions, my feelings told me they were real. It was difficult for my mind to grasp that *my reality* for the last six weeks was not real after all. I felt shell shocked and very fragile.

Kurt was really great. He didn't push me; he would just ask me questions like: "Had the other patients acknowledged that I was in control of the music?" He encouraged me to find out for myself what was real or not. He didn't force me to believe things that I wasn't yet ready to. At first

I wasn't sure what role the nurses had in my stay at the hospital, whether they were good or bad. And were they extensions of Kurt? That was the last major delusion to go. The nurses were simply doing their job; they were there to look after me. Not extensions of Kurt, not evil people controlled by Satan, but just nurses.

As my view of the nurses changed, so did our relationship. I began to appreciate their hard work and the difficult situations they needed to deal with. They had been friends and a great support to Kurt; now they became my friends as well. They had supported me in my illness, now they celebrated with me in my recovery.

That Monday, one day after coming out of the psychosis, nurses urged me to take the next step in my recovery process. In the psychiatric ward there was a Phase system of increased freedom and responsibility. Since entering hospital I had been on Phase I, meaning I basically had no freedom. Each Monday at the community meeting patients would have the opportunity to request an upgrade to the next Phase. The nurses strongly encouraged me to request Phase II. In this Phase I could wear clothes, go for walks with fellow patients, and apply for weekend passes to go home.

I was encouraged that the nurses felt I was ready for Phase II, yet I was also extremely nervous. What if my request was denied; I might be stuck in hospital forever. I could scarcely believe it when they accepted my request. It was one small step towards getting out of hospital. I felt excited and proud. After 6 weeks it was wonderful to actually wear some of my own clothes rather than a hospital gown. Also getting my contacts back again, and actually being able to see, made me feel more myself as well. Nurses and patients looked so different than what I had imagined.

That afternoon I was able to go with other patients on a short walk. I felt like a bird being let out of a cage, wonderfully free. Except for the times I had escaped, it was the first time in six weeks I had gotten any fresh air. (If the air in downtown Vancouver can be considered fresh). It was an exhilarating feeling yet I also felt rather insecure. This was outside of the safe, controlled environment I was used to.

As we walked, the nurse on duty kept glancing my way as if concerned I might try to run away. This was quite amusing to me, as I would now be much too afraid to leave the other patients and venture out alone. I felt much too vulnerable, like a chick freshly hatched from its safe shell. Whereas the hospital seemed like a very dangerous place to me when I was psychotic, as I began to head down the road to recovery, its walls were a place of safety where I would be protected. Although in the hospital I felt well enough, I realized that out in the real world, I would have felt very sick and out of place.

I hadn't gone far on our walk that day until I felt the affect of many weeks of inactivity. My muscles were very weak; I was completely out of shape. Walking just a few blocks completely tired me out.

Over the next several days, I realized that my physical muscles were not the only part of me that felt weak. My sense of identity and trust in my abilities as a rational thinking person were completely shaken. I felt not only the need to earn the trust of others, but also to earn my own trust as well. At one of the community meetings we needed to staple some pages together. I remember the nurse handing me the stapler, and feeling as if she didn't quite trust me with it, like a child who has been allowed to use a knife for the first time. I wasn't even confident that physically I was strong enough to use it.

So, although I was extremely grateful to have come out of the psychosis, the after affects had left me very vulnerable emotionally and mentally. It was difficult for me to deal with the reality that I had been *mentally ill*. Rather than the world around me going crazy, as I had perceived when ill, I had been crazy. There is such a stigma in society about mental illness. Would people I had known and loved before my hospital experience treat me differently? Would they think less of me? I had never given much thought to mental illness in the past. If I had, it would be to think it might happen to other people, but not to me. Now I was forced to come face to face with my ideas of mental illness, how I felt about those who suffered from it…in other words, how I felt about me.

Was the psychotic person I had been the *real me*? If not, if I was in fact the *normal* person from before my illness, would I ever truly recover and feel the same. The psychosis was like a monstrous shadow, a Mr. Hyde, clinging to my sense of self. As I expressed my fears and doubts to Kurt, his words were reassuring, "Dorothy, your psychosis was really no different than when I injured my back and needed medical treatment. Sure, mine was a physical problem and yours had to do with chemicals in your brain, but the psychosis was not your fault. You shouldn't feel bad about it."

I clung to those words. Although I still felt *very bad* about it, logically I knew it was true. There was nothing I could have done personally to either prevent the psychosis from happening or bring myself out of it sooner. Having Kurt support me, rather than reject me for having been mentally ill, helped me to begin to believe in myself again, that I might eventually come out of this experience whole.

Kurt was excited about my continuing improvement; a fragile wife was infinitely better than a crazy one. As the weeks went by, he had wondered if the psychosis would ever end, if I would ever come back. Now, it was if I had come back to life. To him my illness was over. To me, in a way, it was just beginning. Just as a person who has been in an automobile accident ends up physically shaken, cut up, and bruised, I felt shaken, cut up, and bruised on the inside. And yet, my need to become 'normal' again forced me to cover up the emotional cuts and bruises before they even had a chance to heal.

> *Nov. 25—Maintaining improvement. Quite animated and humorous at times. Conversation and group input appropriate. Husband visited—he states that Dorothy is "even better than yesterday"—although she remembers much of her chaotic thoughts and behaviour of a week/month ago—and is very embarrassed.*
>
> *Dorothy is working hard on her autobiography, anxious to complete this and do what's expected, tearful when talking of past events, shows increased affect when discussing her baby, thought processes seem clear. She is inquiring about passes this weekend and would very much like to get home for the weekend.*

I wanted to do everything expected of me to hasten my release from hospital and return my life to normal. To get into phase III, I was required to write an autobiography, answering questions about my family, childhood, and perceptions of my illness. I remember writing that I had a nervous breakdown after losing so much blood following

Martina's birth. I also mentioned dying and coming back, like a near death experience. My having postpartum psychosis just didn't seem to sink in, although Kurt had explained it to me many times. I was on the road to recovery, and definitely not psychotic, but yet in some areas, at certain times, my reason was still a bit clouded.

> *Nov. 26—Patient states feeling really good "like she has woken up." Maintaining improvement, answers appropriately to questions asked, willing to talk about baby and expressed that she can't wait to go home and take care of her baby. Participated in afternoon walk and community meetings. Completed her autobiography.*

Although I was out of the psychosis, the timing of my release was still uncertain. In a sense the hospital still seemed a bit like a prison to me. My release was like climbing an unknown mountain; each phase was a large progression up the hill but could I make it over the top? And upon reaching the top, what would be on the other side? I knew my baby would be there, but it was bittersweet to even think about her, not knowing when it might happen. At this point my hospital experience was still more real to me than Martina. I fully realized now that I had one baby, and that she was a girl. I now had a recent picture of Martina in my room, but I didn't allow myself to think about her too much. To even speculate when I might be able to care for her again was just torturing myself.

At the community meeting that Thursday I requested a weekend pass, a chance to finally get out of hospital for a few days and see what home felt like. I was granted it. Another stepping stone. Sure it would be only for a couple days but it was a start. I would be sleeping in my own bed, not a hospital bed in the psychiatric ward. Little did I realize how much I would wish for that hospital bed before the weekend was over.

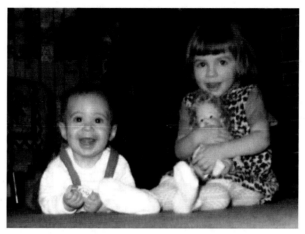

Holding my doll with baby brother George.

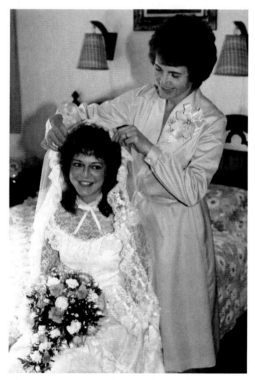

Getting ready—wedding day.

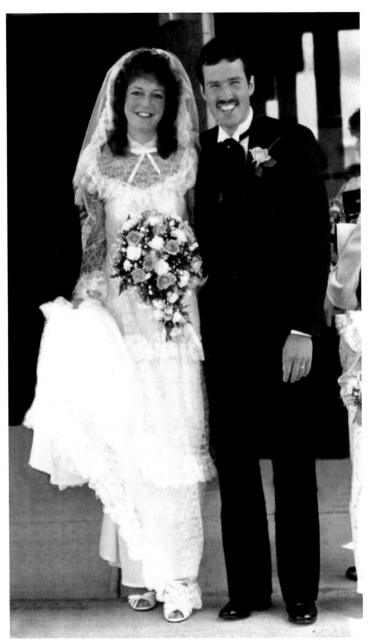

The new Mr. and Mrs. Kurt Ruhwald.

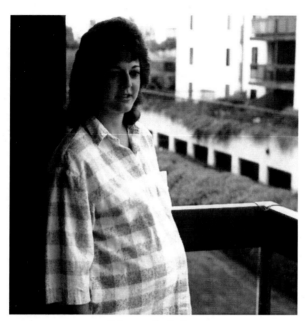

Waiting for baby.

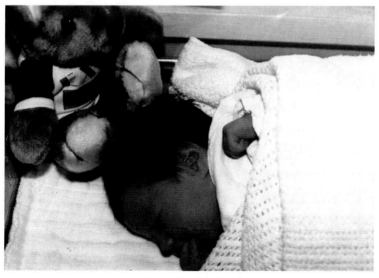

Martina Rose is born.

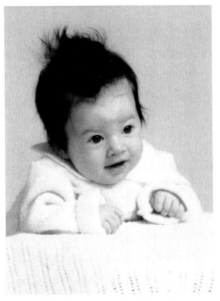

Martina—two months old.

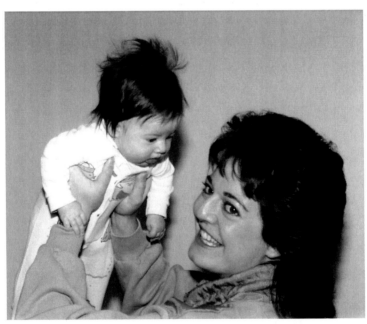

I have my baby back.

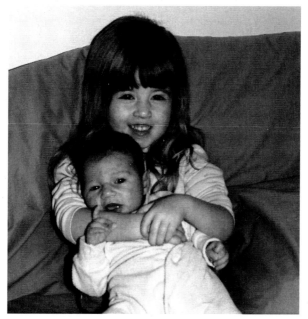

Martina—happy with her baby sister, Natasha Alexis.

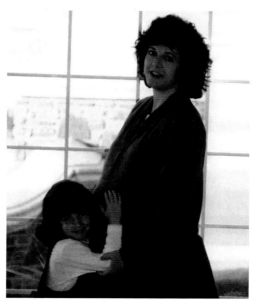

Natasha giving the coming baby a hug.

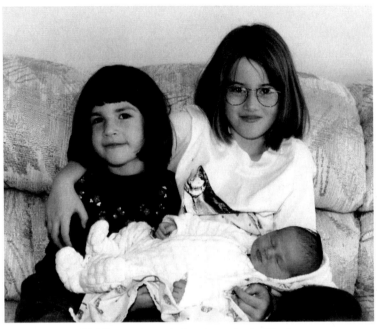

Holding our new baby sister, Sonja Nicole.

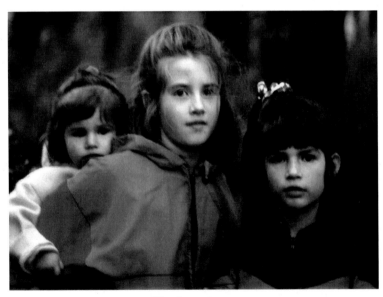

The three sisters.

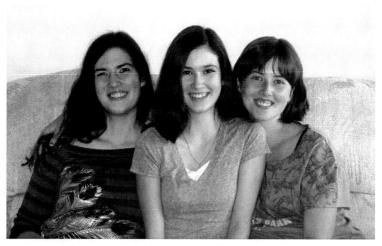

Natasha, Sonja and Martina—my three dreams come true.

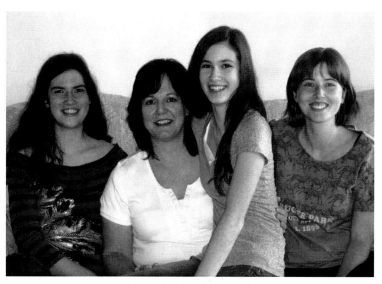

Me and the girls. (2009)

EIGHT

From a Mountain Peak to a Deep Valley

A nticipation and anxiety fought to rule my emotions during the drive home from hospital that Saturday afternoon. Although I was looking forward to finally getting home, if for only a short time, I also felt disorientated. Kurt stopped at a mall to do a bit of shopping. Since we were in the Christmas Season, the stores were extremely crowded. Coming from the ordered environment and security of the hospital, I felt dazed by the busy mall. It was as if I had arrived from a different planet and had culture shock. I felt different from the other people and out-of-place. In a paranoid sort of way I felt that others could tell I wasn't quite normal, that I had just come from hospital. After only a short while, in a near panic, I said, "Kurt, I need to go home! I can't take this anymore!"

Thankfully, he seemed to understand, and we quickly left the store, arriving home as quickly as the busy streets would allow.

Home- yes, it was home but I felt insecure even here, perhaps especially here. My two worlds collided as I entered the apartment. On the one side were memories of the months before the baby's arrival and the first week after she was born. On the other, were the memories of my time in hospital. I was stuck in the middle, not truly belonging in either world.

As I looked into the nursery prepared for Martina I was unable to avoid thinking about her, feeling the emptiness not only in the room, but also in my life as well. Just as we had prepared the room for a baby, so I had prepared my heart for a baby, only to have her torn away. I remembered changing my sweet little baby, putting a beret in her hair (yes, she had that much hair), holding her and rocking her, but it seemed a lifetime away. In a sense my illness was much more real to me than my baby. I had no idea when I would see Martina next. My fear was that I might never be truly *normal* and fit to look after her. It was easier to just keep my distance from that room and any thoughts of Martina.

That first weekend home I didn't do much at all. The anticipation I had felt regarding coming home slowly lost the fight to anxiety. I found it difficult to perform even simple household tasks, such as cooking frozen vegetables.

That evening Kurt and I went for a walk in the neighbourhood and visited my Aunt Helen and Uncle Bob. My contribution to the conversation was practically non-existent; there just didn't seem to be anything to say. I didn't even feel capable of small talk. It was simpler to just let Kurt do the talking. Although I still felt out of place in the real world, it felt good to be among people who weren't working through a mental illness. The walk was the most therapeutic. Just to get outside in the fresh air and forget for a while was a break.

I had hoped to sleep better at home, but that night my sleep was very shallow. At any moment I could open my eyes and feel fully awake. Sometime after midnight a strong feeling of anxiety began building inside of me. My heart was pounding and I found it impossible to settle down and relax. There was no *one* thing that I was afraid of; in fact there was no real reason for me to be afraid. It was just a growing emotion, which I felt helpless to stop. I shook Kurt awake. "Please," I pleaded, "I need to go back to the hospital. I have this terrible fear inside of me! I'm just so scared!"

Kurt tried to reassure me: "You're really OK! Try to wait until morning. If you still want to, then I'll take you back to hospital."

By morning I felt a bit better. At least there was now something I could do to distract myself from the anxiety. The hospital also didn't seem quite so appealing anymore, especially since I knew it would be another week before I could come home again on a weekend pass.

As I showered that morning suicidal thoughts ran through my mind. It's not as if I really wanted to kill myself; these thoughts of hopelessness and dying just seemed to come into my head unbidden: *'It would have been better for everyone if I had bled to death in the delivery room.' 'I'll never be normal again.' 'What kind of wife and mother will I be; I'm just a no-mind.' 'I'll never fit in with normal people.'*

I remember wondering, *'If I kill myself in the state I'm in now, would I go to heaven or hell.'* The thought of hell terrified me. I had experienced it in the last several weeks of psychosis; I didn't want to go through it again.

I had no appetite and felt nauseated. When I held a fork at mealtime it would shake back and forth in my fingers. This was just a side affect of the lithium, which went away after a while. But I didn't realize this at the time; I felt like such a hopeless case.

That afternoon as Kurt watched the Grey Cup football game on TV I lay beside him on the couch. I was oblivious to the game but at least I could take some comfort from Kurt's physical presence.

As we passed the nurses station on our arrival back in hospital a nurse called out, "Dorothy, how was your weekend home?"

"Well, it went OK until last night…then I felt really panicked and anxious." I replied somewhat sheepishly.

"For the first time home it was maybe a bit too long." And inside I had to agree. I was glad, though, that I didn't come crawling back in the middle of the night. That would have made me feel like I had somehow failed.

In a way it was a relief to be back in hospital. Sure, it was boring, but at least it was safe and secure. It was also predictable; I knew exactly what to expect every hour of the day.

During that first weekend home I had plunged from feeling better and more completely myself every day into a severe depression. My previous feelings of depression were from gaining a few pounds or having a blue day but this was a completely different animal altogether. It was as if I was being crushed by a heavy weight, making me slow and sluggish. I felt dark and dead inside, and emotionally numb, incapable of feeling anything: love, happiness, even sadness—only depression. Laughing, and even crying, seemed beyond my capabilities.

Mentally, my thought processes seemed to be so slow; concentration was difficult. As much as my brain seemed to have sped up during the manic phase of my illness, it was now on the opposite spectrum. I felt brain damaged; even my memory was affected. Although I had memorized many verses from my Bible, they had all vanished from my memory. My symptoms only caused my already strong feelings of dread and anxiety to build. I felt completely unable to cope.

Although going through a psychosis and being separated from Martina could make me *feel* depressed, I believe the major cause of my depression was biochemical. It just seemed to arrive from nowhere. I found it very frightening. How could I even begin to deal with this?

When I attempted to explain my feelings to a nurse she said, "Oh, this is probably Baby Blues or postpartum depression... It's quite normal and will go away after a while."

Postpartum psychosis, then postpartum depression? It will go away after a while? Somehow I didn't find her answer reassuring, in the least! How could she so confidently tell me it would go away after *a while*? She wasn't in my shoes. After the psychosis ended I felt at least somewhat well, now I was sick in a completely different way.

The patients were more helpful. As I shared my feelings at a small group meeting they gave me more than sympathy and pat answers. They gave me empathy and understanding. Many were either struggling with depression or had worked through one in the past. When they told me things would get better, I listened. In contrast to the nurses, they *were* in my shoes.

> *Dec. 1—Dorothy's mood continues to be depressed, is frustrated with this low mood. Short evening passes have been approved so Dorothy can go out with husband.*

That evening Kurt took me for a drive to Stanley Park. For that hour or so I could just forget my feelings, and not think. I felt relaxed and peaceful inside. I would have liked to just go on driving forever, far away from the hospital and my whole postpartum experience.

> *Slightly tearful during conversation. Querying if poor concentration was permanent—accepted reassurance that it was part of illness right now.*

At one time my anxiety and restlessness were so severe that I would walk from my room to the lounge, then to the TV room, over and over again. My sister Marie phoned; I talked for a couple minutes, then abruptly said, "I'm sorry, I just can't talk right now…and hung up." Then back to the pacing again. But nothing seemed to help; I just couldn't shake the awful feeling of dread and anxiety inside.

> *Dec. 4—Appeared to be brighter today. Stated looking forward to going home for*

weekend, she hoped that it would be less stressful this weekend. Participated in group meetings giving compliments to people on the ward. Participated in afternoon walk. Conversations remain appropriate with patients and staff.

On one afternoon walk we passed by a school. Children were playing outside. I remember thinking, with a heavy feeling inside, 'Soon Martina will be going to school.' Of course that was really stretching it, as she was only a couple of months old at the time. But then I really had no idea when I would get out of hospital or see her again. Even when I was released would I be able to look after her? A lot of the patients at hospital seemed very normal, more so than I, yet they were still here. And even after being released, some patients still came to hospital on an outpatient basis. I wondered: 'Would I need to come back on an outpatient basis or possibly live in a group home for a while?' There was just no way for me to know. To compare myself to other patients was not really productive because a lot of them had psychological problems that they needed to work through before they left hospital, whereas with me it was biochemical. There was nothing psychological about it; it was more like just waiting to recover from an illness. I hadn't talked to the nurses about what I might expect; perhaps I was afraid to ask. There was not much communication with my psychiatrist at that time either.

The nurses talked to me about possibly having Martina come in hospital, having me care for her in my room. The thought of seeing Martina again, not to mention caring for her again was enough to lift my spirits, to give me some hope. Yet, I also had reservations; was I ready? I had no doubts about my natural ability to care for her, yet I didn't feel quite strong enough yet.

That evening, at home on my weekend pass, Kurt and I discussed having Martina room in with me. We also phoned Kurt's parents in Victoria, and talked about it with them. The thought of Martina staying in the psychiatric ward with me upset them greatly. They were very concerned about her safety.

When I first heard their reaction it angered me. This was my baby after all, not theirs. Yet I knew their strong emotions stemmed from a great love for Martina, whom they had cherished these last several weeks. Looking at the situation from their end, I realized a psychiatric ward would not be my first choice for my baby either. It wasn't so much that I was concerned about Martina's safety. In the right circumstances I knew a baby would bring so much joy to those on the psychiatric ward. But it was not at all set up for the care of a baby. Where would she sleep? How would I heat up milk for her in the middle of the night? And speaking of nights, I was not yet sleeping well. What would waking up every three hours do to my already fragile state of mind?

After discussing the situation at length, I felt very peaceful about our decision to leave Martina in Victoria with Kurt's parents until my release from hospital. She was being well cared for, and I needed this extra time to recover.

Although I would not be seeing Martina again for some time, talking and thinking about her brought her closer to me. I didn't know when, but I had hope that it would definitely happen. I just needed to be patient a while longer. That seed of hope gave me the strength I needed to continue on the road to recovery.

That weekend I ventured out to do some grocery shopping with Kurt and even prepared a batch of our family's traditional Christmas cookie dough. It would be a long time until I would be comfortable out shopping, and the weekend was not free from fear, but yes, it was definitely an improvement from last time. And just doing those couple *normal* activities comforted me and encouraged me. I *could* accomplish something worthwhile.

> *Dec. 6, evening—Returned from pass accompanied by husband—both report that this weekend was better than last—that "home" is more therapeutic than hospital.*

NINE

The Road Home

Monday morning in the community meeting, I again applied for, and received, the next phase. Being in phase III meant I could now leave the hospital with a patient on phase IV or a responsible adult (I guess that would be Kurt). It also meant I could begin working towards my discharge from hospital.

I didn't know what would all have to take place before I could go home; I just tried to do what was expected. I knew the nurses thought my visiting with other patients in the lounge was positive, so I made sure I spent plenty of time there. My thinking was: 'They'll think I'm recovering, I'll get better 'marks' on my hospital records, and I might get released sooner.'

Time spent in the patient's lounge was positive for other reasons as well. Visiting with others kept my mind occupied. My own room seemed so cold and empty. I felt more comfortable around other people. Television was even difficult for me to concentrate on; in the patient's lounge I could talk or listen, as I felt comfortable. On one occasion I asked a few other patients to play Ping-Pong with me downstairs. The ball bounced on the floor more often than the table but we had a great time laughing at each other. And that was so important—to be able to laugh again, for whatever reason.

Although my depression did continue, day by day I began to feel a little better, a bit more able to function. It was as if I was taking baby steps toward wellness. When Kurt took me out to a restaurant for hot chocolate one evening I was actually able to make small talk. This really made me feel good, because even days earlier small talk would have been impossible for me, especially in a public place. I actually felt almost like a *normal* person while out with Kurt.

When I was first depressed my emotions seemed to be dried up; I couldn't laugh or cry. Now, they gradually began to come back. In one group session with other patients we were asked to tell our proudest moment. I shared with the group how very proud I felt holding Martina in my arms immediately after her birth. The tears finally came. In another group I found myself laughing when a patient told how he had seen Jesus bartending downtown. Others had laughed at the crazy things I had said; now it was my turn. Many *funny* things are said and done on a psychiatric ward; it was natural for patients to laugh at each other. It wasn't a critical, belittling thing. It was finding humour, and grabbing that burst of joy that goes with it, in a place where there wasn't generally a lot of joy.

An event that encouraged me further to believe I was heading down the road to recovery was my participation in our Wednesday night supper. In hospital, each Wednesday, a group of patients would cook the evening meal. All patients were then free to invite family or guests to enjoy it with them. This was a special time of the week. Being in charge of the meal included deciding the menu (we were on a set budget), shopping for the food required, and preparing the meal. This week it was my group's turn. After much discussion we decided to make Chilli, with French Bread and Salad. The afternoon before the big event, we all walked to the store to buy the necessary ingredients. As we walked, one woman, Maggie, wasn't watching where she was going. Looking straight ahead, she walked right into a huge puddle. It was hilarious, at least to us; we just couldn't stop laughing. People passing by must have thought we were nuts, but since we technically were, it didn't matter. It was just so wonderful to laugh freely again after so long.

I found the actual shopping very stressful, especially figuring out what we could get for the money we had. After what seemed like a very long time, for such a small amount of groceries, we managed to buy everything we needed and returned to hospital.

> *Dec. 8—Dorothy continues improvement. During 1:1 expressing concern that she may not recover completely. "I'm still not back to my normal personality" States concentration is often a problem " I would like to get back into my own routine at home."*

The next evening we made our Chilli. The dinner went very well; the chilli actually tasted very good. I had considered myself quite an accomplished cook (being taught that the way to a man's heart is through his stomach) but after being sick this humble meal was a big deal to me. I felt very proud, especially to have Kurt come and share it with me. It was another small but important accomplishment.

> *Dec. 9—Dorothy did an excellent job cooking Wed. night meal and organizing the dinner "set-up." She is anxious to discuss discharge with Dr., feeling she is ready to leave hospital.*

The hospital routine when I was psychotic had seemed very busy, more than I could keep up with. Now I found it boring, stagnating. I just wanted to go home and get on with my life. To help fill my time I found projects to do. I worked on Thank-you cards for Martina's baby gifts. This sounds like a simple task but it was very difficult for me. My writing was shaky, with many spelling mistakes. It was almost as if I needed to learn to write all over again. Although I was able to complete only a few cards a day, they did finally get done, giving me a great sense of accomplishment.

I also brought some embroidery from home to work on in my free hours. At first I didn't have the attention span to spend more than a few minutes sewing, but gradually that improved. Although I used to just love reading books, at this stage in my recovery it was impossible. I would read the first page over and over but the words would just not sink in.

Our daily walks were an event I looked forward to each day, a small taste of freedom. Each day I would head out, even in the rain. I had learned that an umbrella was very necessary in Vancouver. Although I still felt different from people passing by, the outside world was beginning to feel more comfortable.

One day I went for a walk with Maggie, a fellow patient. Although Maggie was old enough to be my mother, she was a real friend. In a way she was like a mother to me while I was in hospital. That day we picked up some bread from the patient's kitchen and walked to English Bay to feed the geese. The sense of freedom and independence was exhilarating. And although I had been afraid our poor sense of direction would get us lost, we made it back to hospital, safe and sound.

Those walks were very special. We were different ages, some male and some female, with completely different problems, from eating disorders to manic-depressive illness, but we all shared a certain bond. This bond, our shared hospital experience, allowed us to feel comfortable with each other and just be ourselves. In a way we were like a huge mismatched family.

I found that although my days could be filled with walks and other busyness, nights were still difficult. I would have loved to fill them with sleep. Peaceful sleep would have been nice, but I would have taken sleep in any form. Before my illness, I had never had trouble sleeping. Now, it just seemed to elude me. Although I must have slept some time during the night, it was very shallow. I seemed to be in a state of semi-consciousness. At any time I could open my eyes and feel wide-awake. This concerned me a great deal, as I knew that sleep deprivation was hardly conducive to a healthy mind. I did take sleeping pills for a few days but since I was afraid of becoming dependent on them and they only gave me a couple of hours sound sleep anyway, I soon quit.

Now that I was on Phase III, I had the increased responsibility of a buddy. A buddy would be a patient just new to the ward, who I could show around, take to meetings, and just generally, be a *buddy* to. My first buddy that I was assigned was an uncooperative type, like I had been on first arriving. He did not want to be shown to meetings, let alone leave his bed. It made me empathize with the person who might have been unlucky enough to get me as a buddy.

My next buddy was a woman I'll call Mary. I still clearly remember the night she came in. Since it was getting close to Christmas, the patients had been busy decorating a tree outside of the patient's lounge. I was sitting in that lounge when Mary came in. She chatted for a while, sharing how she had planned to do some singing in a choir at church for Christmas. She then proceeded to demonstrate. Mary sang *Oh Holy Night*. She had a wonderful, powerful voice. Although I have heard that song sung many times, it was never as meaningful as when I heard it that night. Sung by one hurting person to a whole roomful of hurting people. Nurses gathered in the lounge. When Mary had finished we all sang *Silent Night*. It was beautiful to be singing a song about *calm* and *quiet* and *heavenly peace*, in a place where it was so desperately needed. But did God actually care about the state of our minds? I just wasn't sure. My faith in God, which I had always assumed was so strong, was as shaken and fragile as my emotional health.

One other patient, although not positive, sticks in my mind as well. She had just been admitted. I didn't at first notice any reason why she might need to be in hospital. However, one day as we were both sitting in the patient's lounge, she looked over at me and just kept staring. She called me *darling daughter*, not taking her gaze off me for a second. I asked her, "Do you think I'm your daughter?"

Another patient told me, "Just ignore her!"—yet I couldn't. Her behaviour intrigued me. She was obviously psychotic, and I wondered if that frighteningly crazy look which I saw in her eyes had been in mine. I wanted to know what she was thinking and what was going on inside her head. I didn't want to back down. In a way it was like looking at my illness and I wanted to understand it, to understand her.

Trying to understand and sympathize with someone who is psychotic is not always the wisest idea, though. She began leaning towards me, talking in a menacing way. Perhaps seeing in my eyes that I was not afraid bothered her. It took several nurses to finally force her to leave the patient's lounge. I was left with a very unsettled feeling inside, as if I had been looking back at myself only a few weeks previously. Although much of my memory of my psychosis was gone, I did remember believing that several patients were my children as well.

I was starting to get very anxious to find out when I

might leave hospital so I made an appointment with my Doctor. When I went in for the appointment I was quite nervous as I hadn't spoken to him for several weeks and was sure I'd have to come up with many reasons why I felt I was well enough to leave. Surprisingly, the first thing he said to me was "So, when do you want to go home?"

"Tomorrow… right away!" I stammered. I just couldn't believe it was truly going to happen. I was shocked that he would actually set a release date without talking to me about how I was feeling and discussing my progress. I suppose that since the nurses reported to him very regularly he felt knowledgeable enough to make the decision. Obviously the nurses felt I was now ready to be released.

We set the following Tuesday, Dec. 15, as my release date. I felt just wonderful, like I had received a million dollars. Besides a date for my release, the Dr. gave me a different gift as well, a new hope. We discussed my having more children. Since coming out of the psychosis I hadn't even considered it an option. There was no way I felt I could risk going through another psychosis. He listened patiently to my fears, and then said, "You know, Dorothy… I wouldn't tell you not to have more children. There is a one in three chance a psychosis would happen after another birth. But, now that we know lithium works for you, we could put you on it at the first sign of any symptoms."

I pondered those words as I left his office. Sure, there

was still a risk, but I knew it wouldn't be anywhere near as bad if I was successfully treated right away. I still wasn't sure I was willing to accept that risk, especially not in the near future, but at least I now had that choice.

As I walked past the nurses' station a huge smile broke out on my face; I was really going home! It was obvious by the smug expressions on the nurses' faces that they had known about my release even before my appointment. They were very happy for me, but then my release was a success for them as well.

One nurse cautioned, "Dorothy, it won't be over once you leave here." Wise words, which I would remember often in the upcoming months. But for now, I wanted to just enjoy the thought of finally going home.

We made plans for the days following my discharge from hospital. When I was able, I would go to Kurt's parents' home in Victoria. I would stay till I felt comfortable looking after Martina on my own, and then bring her home with me. An appointment was also made for me with the Mental Health Office near our home. I would be under the care of a psychiatrist until I went off lithium.

Dec. 10—Dorothy took the initiative today to set a discharge date with Dr. G____ (next Tuesday) Affect bright and more animated. Dorothy states she feels far from her "normal" *but is improving daily. Optimistic outlook regarding discharge.*

I was still concerned about my not sleeping well as the Doctor had said it was important for me to get good sleep. The nurses reassured me that sleep would come in time, and not to worry about it.

Although I was really looking forward to leaving the hospital, I was somewhat anxious about leaving my safe predictable haven. I knew I would also miss the other patients. Having gone through the crisis of mental illness together was a special bond.

It was also very difficult to see other patients get more ill even as I was getting better. I watched as one patient left the hospital to get electric shock treatment. Mary, my buddy, went from being, at least to me, quite normal, to a bundle of anxiety. She had a white, sweaty face, and a terrible look of anxiety, fear and panic in her eyes. And there was nothing I could do to help her. Yet I knew I couldn't let her illness hamper my own recovery. I needed to concentrate on my own health. My focus needed to be my upcoming release and finally seeing Martina again. Martina… the pot of gold at the end of a not so promising rainbow. Just thinking about her renewed my optimism. One day left after this weekend home and I'd be free!

TEN

A Family Reunited

The weekend home passed quickly. It was as if my mind and body were both straining forwards to my discharge date on Tuesday. I felt like a graduation student, reviewing my time in school with other students.

Along with the bad, I also had so many good memories: a doctor dancing a jig with a middle-aged female patient, laughing over a game of Ping-Pong, a patient playing the guitar and singing. These all added up to make my hospital experience not only the most terrifying of my life but also one of the most special and enlightening times as well. Now that I was leaving I felt almost privileged to have experienced life in the psychiatric ward.

Normally I would not have associated with people in a psychiatric ward; I would have been turned off by the way they looked or acted. Now, after having experienced mental illness firsthand, I could look beyond their illness and see the very special, strong people that they were.

> *Dec. 14—Maintains improvement, talking about appropriate discharge concerns, she appears to have priorities in order, somewhat concerned whether in laws will trust she is now well enough to trust with the baby, her thinking is optimistic about her ability to cope.*

It was so wonderful to know I was finally going home! A girl came to my room and congratulated me, saying, "Now, don't get sick again. Get out and stay out!"

Well, that was definitely my plan. I may have appreciated the positives of my hospital stay but I had no desire to ever visit a psychiatric ward as a patient again. And yet, even as I was thrilled to be leaving hospital, there was hesitation as well. I felt a real sense of beginning again, of learning all over again. What would the future hold for me? Although I was considered well enough to leave hospital, I was still far from my *normal* self. My mind still felt very dull and slow, as if I was moving at a different pace from the rest of the world. Would I continue to improve? Would this depression and sluggishness ever leave? I longed for the time when I could finally say, "Yes, I feel completely well again. I feel like the same person I was before I got sick."

But no one was able to tell me when that day would come, if ever. I knew I just needed to press on, working with the *me* I had, and concentrate on my role as wife and mother.

> *Dec. 15—Dorothy attended both elective groups today "I want to learn as much as possible before leaving" affect bright—anxious about how she will do at home but hopeful. Follow up Dec. 21ˢᵗ. with Richmond Mental Health. GP notified of discharge. Discharged at 1700 hrs.*

I had fought to escape the hospital in my psychosis, and worked towards leaving from the moment I regained my sanity. The big moment had finally arrived. And like so many such occasions, it turned out to be a bit of an anticlimax. There was no fanfare as I walked out of hospital with Kurt carrying my suitcase. And yet, having the knowledge that I was free, from hospital and from the worst of my illness, made even the everyday sounds of city traffic music to my ears.

My first project upon returning home was replenishing

the refrigerator. Kurt took me for a quick trip for groceries, and although being out in public was getting easier, I still felt a bit uncomfortable and out of place. Whatever I did, whether being out in public, or at home, I struggled with a vague dull, heavy feeling of dread.

Little tasks that I would normally not have given a thought to, I now used to gauge my improvement—how I felt when out grocery shopping, how difficult it was to cook meals, or to do a load of laundry. It was one small way I could concretely measure my improvement. Even though I still felt depressed, knowing that I had found it easier to do the dishes that day, for instance, than the day before, gave me some hope of further recovery.

The day after I was released from hospital, Kurt bought a Christmas tree. That evening he put the lights on, and then since he needed to attend a meeting, asked me to finish decorating it. "Don't you realize there's no way I can do such a big job?" I retorted.

Seemingly with total confidence in my ability, he shot back, "Sure you can. Just work at it slowly!"

"Sure I can, ha!" I mumbled. "It's easy for you to say." But yet somehow Kurt's confidence encouraged me to at least try. So I kept plugging away at it. It was far from enjoyable. This was the first time in several months that I was completely alone. The apartment seemed so empty and lonely. Even music playing in the background didn't dispel the gloomy feeling I had inside. But I was accomplishing what, to me, had seemed an overwhelming job. When Kurt arrived home the decorations were all up and I had one more achievement to feel good about.

We had decided that I would take the trip to see Martina the next day, Thursday. So before Kurt left for work, he dropped me off at the Ferry Terminal. I really appreciated that he trusted me enough to take the trip myself. It was a big deal to me—a real challenge. I felt sort of like a little girl allowed to go on a bus trip by herself for the first time. After several months of having my freedom restricted, although legitimately, I didn't have much confidence in my ability to cope on my own in the outside world. Knowing that Kurt did have confidence in me helped a lot.

I was really excited about seeing Martina again. On the other hand I was feeling a bit nervous and unsure. What kind of a reception would I get from my in-laws? Would they treat me differently now?

I need not have worried. When I arrived in Victoria, my mother-in-law greeted me with a big hug. "I'm so glad you're better," she said, "and finally able to care for Martina." Her words also gave me confidence, as if she didn't doubt my abilities.

Kurt's mom had left Martina at home in the care of her Opa. Although I was disappointed that Martina was not with her, the drive to their home went very quickly. My mom-in-law chatted non-stop about Martina—how sweet she was, the new things she was learning to do. I had a building sense of excitement and anticipation as we drove towards their home. I was truly going to see my baby again.

As the car pulled up into the driveway, my heart began to beat faster. I wiped my sweating palms on my pants. *This was it!* Upon entering the house, I noticed Kurt's Dad painfully making his way down the stairs, with a bundle in his arms. He was quite ill, yet he made the extra effort to bring Martina *to me*. I met them halfway up the stairs. My father-in-law put Martina into my waiting arms. Without uttering a word, his actions said to me: '*We have carried Martina for a few steps in her life, now we give her back to you!*' It was a very symbolic and emotional moment for me, as weeping, I carried Martina up the stairs.

My *mother's* heart was very happy to claim Martina again, to hold her, and look into her expressive round eyes. Yet in the back of my mind was a subtle disappointment. My tiny newborn was gone. In its place was a chubby little character that smiled and cooed. Although Martina at almost three months was wonderful, she was hardly the same baby I remembered. I knew babies change so much in the first three months yet I hadn't realized how much. It hit me hard... there was so much I had missed. Although I was very grateful to care for her again, I also felt cheated.

I didn't know how Martina would relate to me after so

many weeks of separation. To my great relief, she didn't make strange at all. I remember holding her up in the air and getting her to laugh. My mother-in-law said, "Oh, we've never gotten her to laugh like that!"

Somehow, that statement reassured me. Perhaps the very strong bond I shared with Martina following her birth was still there, just waiting to be renewed. We just needed time to get to know each other again.

Kurt's parents were both very good about not interfering, and just giving Martina up to me completely. They told me her schedule, and then left everything to me. I didn't feel awkward with Martina at all. However, I did feel a strong desire to make up for lost time. In my eyes, part of a mother's role was being the central figure in her baby's life. I needed time to become that again.

The first night Kurt's mother fed Martina when she woke up, to give me a chance to sleep. I had been concerned about waking up with a baby during the night. I wasn't sleeping well to begin with. What affect would night feedings have on my already poor sleeping patterns? By the second night, I was willing to give it a try. Although I didn't sleep too soundly after feeding Martina, to my great relief, my total night's sleep was generally the same.

On Saturday, Kurt's parents accompanied me on the ferry back to Vancouver. On the trip back, a group of Asian girls crowded around Martina, oohing, and aahing over how beautiful she was. With her huge eyes, and thick head of black hair, she looked just like a doll, and I was very proud to be her mother.

Within a very short time of our arrival back at our apartment, Kurt's parents left, perhaps realizing this new family needed time to be alone together again. The nursery now had a baby sleeping in it; our family was once more complete.

I found it surprisingly easy to adjust to having a baby to look after. Martina was just a wonderful baby to have around, so happy and contented. My parents phoned to see how things were going. I told them, "God knew what I would have to go through after Martina's birth. Maybe He gave me such an extra special baby, sort of as a consolation prize... it would be so much worse to have to go through a psychosis and not have anything to show for it. At least I have a wonderful little baby to care for and keep me busy."

At the first opportunity, Kurt and I took a whole roll of pictures—Martina by herself, Martina with Mom, and Martina with Dad. When these pictures were developed I was very relieved to see that in the pictures I actually looked like a normal person and mother. That meant a great deal to me. Even if I didn't feel like myself on the inside at least my outward appearance didn't show that I had been crazy and was now depressed.

The first Sunday home together we all went to church

for a special Christmas Cantata. Kurt really enjoyed it and no doubt it was very good. But I just didn't have the attention span or concentration to sit through it all. I was only too happy to have the excuse of a fussing baby to keep me pacing out in the foyer.

I felt very awkward the first few Sundays back in church. My name had been in the bulletin for several weeks requesting prayer for *postpartum depression*. Well, what I had suffered went way beyond typical postpartum depression. So I didn't know what people knew about my illness, if anything at all, or how they felt towards me. Being so new in town, I also didn't know people well enough to open up to them. I didn't want to be rejected so I retreated behind a wall of reserve so I couldn't be hurt. I also felt quite numb anyway from the depression and didn't feel capable of holding a conversation with anyone that I didn't know well. So I just allowed Kurt to do the talking.

People would sometimes ask me the typical "How are you doing?" I would answer "Fine." After all, I didn't know if they were just asking to be polite or if they *really* wanted to know how I was doing. What did bother me was when people in the congregation would ask Kurt how I was doing in my hearing. I might be five feet away, yet they acted like I didn't exist. In a way it was understandable; they were probably unsure whether I wanted to talk about it. I really wouldn't have minded; that is, if I was sure they really wanted to know because they cared.

Possibly I didn't seem that approachable at that time either. If I had gone through a physical illness I'm sure people would have felt quite comfortable asking me about it but mental illness is a scary subject. People seem to pretend it just doesn't exist or could never touch their own lives.

Especially because I felt somewhat uncomfortable around our church family, it was extra special to be invited to Kurt's cousins Edgar and Heather's home, for that Christmas Eve. I knew they had visited me when I was psychotic, although I had no memory of that time. Heather had also visited me in the psychiatric ward after I had come out of the psychosis. Throughout everything, they had remained supportive, not only to me, but also to Kurt. It was so important to have that unconditional acceptance.

Christmas day we went to Edgar's parents' home to share Christmas Day with them. Once again, it was very nice to be included. No one really talked of my having been ill, aside from the usual "How are YOU?" but I felt that they really cared. They didn't need to invite us to join their family yet they made that extra effort on a Christmas where we would have otherwise felt quite lonely and isolated. That meant a lot to both Kurt and myself.

Although my thinking faculties were pretty much in order, I in one instance that afternoon had a *blip* in my rational thinking. There was a conversation about typing taking place. I piped up, "Did you know there is a new type-writer being invented that follows the alphabet, instead of having the letters as they are now on a typewriter."

There was silence in the room; Kurt looked at me rather doubtfully. But it was true. I *had* remembered my brother Peter telling me about it. After further thought, it hit me. It was a memory of a phone conversation with my brother during my psychosis, not exactly reliable, nor even reality. I felt just sick; like I could sink into the floor.

ELEVEN

A New Year, Search for Answers

*A*fter Christmas I settled into a regular routine of caring for Martina, cooking, and cleaning. This *routine* did keep me busy. But after being in hospital, almost always surrounded by other people, I found myself quite lonely. Kurt was naturally often at work. Martina was excellent company—I don't know what I would have done without her cheerful presence. But I longed for other women to talk to, especially someone who could understand how I was feeling.

My sister, Marie, came to visit me in January with her daughter. Because I had talked with her quite often on the phone while in hospital, I felt comfortable now talking with her about my hospital experience. I did wonder, however, if she felt that I was my *normal self* or did she see a difference in me. Before Marie left, I overheard Kurt ask her if *she* thought I was back to normal. I felt so angry; why didn't he just ask me?

Even as anger boiled inside of me, I realized it was a question in my mind as well, yet to actually voice it would have been too threatening. My sense of identity was still too fragile to risk a negative answer.

It was difficult for me to discuss how I was feeling with Kurt. I knew that in his eyes I was basically well. And considering my condition just weeks earlier I *was* doing great. How could I blame him if he wanted to put the last few months behind him and get on with life? Didn't I want to do exactly the same? Yet part of me needed to review and assimilate the last few months into my life, to come to terms with them.

There was a postpartum depression support group in the Vancouver area but since my experience was not a *typical* postpartum depression, I didn't think they could possibly understand me. They could certainly have offered support for the depression I was now experiencing, but the psychosis part of my illness was what I felt I most needed empathy with. I would have loved to talk with someone who had personally gone through Postpartum Psychosis but there was no one available.

My parents phoned often to see how I was feeling. They spoke quite openly about my being depressed, yet I still felt somewhat hesitant to talk about it. There was still that part of me that wanted to forget about my whole postpartum illness, to somehow ignore it and hope it just went away on its own. I also didn't want to burden my family with my feelings of depression.

Counseling at this time would perhaps have been beneficial, yet I likely would have denied the need for it. Wouldn't that be a sign of weakness, a sign that there was still something *wrong* with me?

A health nurse did stop by the apartment to check on Martina and I. Yet again, I felt this need to convince her I was really OK. Sure, I might be feeling somewhat depressed and not yet 100%, but it wasn't anything I couldn't handle myself.

I also visited the Mental Health Clinic regularly. The nurse was very caring yet I sensed both the nurse and psychiatrist didn't quite understand my past illness. I was in a category somewhere between postpartum depression and manic-depression or schizophrenia. I was hesitant to talk in a negative way about my feelings. Every word was being analyzed for their all too familiar medical records. If I appeared emotionally unstable or sick, would I be sent back to hospital? Even though I felt a strong need to really be honest about my experience and feelings, in my eyes, the risk was too great.

It would have been easier to open up to the nurse and psychiatrist if they would have approached my illness a bit differently. Psychotherapy was not needed. What I did need was someone to understand and acknowledge the suffering and pain caused by a psychotic experience. Someone to say, "It's normal for your identity to be completely shaken up, for you to question not only yourself but the foundation of your beliefs. After all, you've been through an emotional and mental earthquake."

Yet, what I received was the attitude, "Let's fix you and get rid of your negative feelings…" rather than, "You have every right to be hurt and afraid!"

Not only was I feeling the effects of an emotional and mental earthquake, I was feeling very shaken up spiritually as well. Although I had been a Christian since I was five years old, up until this point, I had never had my faith really tested. I found myself re-evaluating my whole belief system. I had always believed that God was in control of my life. After being psychotic, could I even believe there was a God? If there was a God how could he allow this to happen, not just to me, but to anyone? How could I *trust* him now? What kind of a God was He anyway?

Crazy religious thoughts were so common during my psychosis. What did they all mean, if anything? I struggled with the question: did Satan cause my psychosis or did God cause/allow it?

In a psychosis, you have no control over your mind. All you know is what you're feeling and experiencing. Therefore you have nothing to logically reason with. You can't say, "Well, I'm going through a hard time. I'm sick but I know God is with me." In my psychosis God seemed miles away, yet I felt Satan breathing down my neck. As a Christian I had been taught that God's presence would never leave me, yet I felt that God had *forsaken* me, at least during my psychosis.

I had also seen a side of God that I had never seen before—a God who would allow everything to be taken away from me, even my rational mind. To me, it was as if God was saying to me: *"You will believe and follow me if you have church, friends, family, and your baby, but will you still follow me if everything is taken away from you? Are you willing to truly put me first, truly make me Lord of your life?"*

I searched the Bible for answers. It seemed that God was ready for my questions.

> *"As you do now know the path of the wind, or*
> *how the body is formed in a mother's womb,*
> *so you cannot understand the work of God,*
> *the Maker of all things."* (Ecclesiastes 11:5)

OK. I could accept that, so long as God knew what He was doing! I felt a bit like Peter who said in *John 6:68* ."..*to whom shall we go? You have the words of eternal life.*" I knew that God might ask more than I felt capable of giving, but He was the only one I could turn to.

I began attending a Moms and Tots group at our church. They were doing a Bible Study on Daniel. It was quite a 'coincidence' that we studied the passage where God caused King Nebuchadnezzar to become insane. So there was somewhere in the Bible where psychosis (insanity) was at least mentioned. I was very interested to study these passages when I got home and discover what could be learned from them. The following verses were especially of interest to me:

> *Daniel 4: 31-33 (It dealt with King Nebuchadnezzar's madness, his symptoms.)*
>
> *: 34 (After a time, his sanity was restored.)*
>
> *: 35 "He does as He pleases...No one can hold back his hand or say to him: 'What have you done?'"*
>
> *: 36 (King Nebuchadnezzar not only recovered, but he became even greater than before!)*
>
> *: 37 "...everything He does is right and all His ways are just."*

What really jumped out at me from these verses was that King Nebuchadnezzar's illness was for a specific time period, after which he was not only restored to health again but he became even greater than before. So his illness was not simply an arbitrary act by an uncaring God but was part of a plan for his life to bring about changes. God definitely showed the king that He was in control of his life. What I found especially encouraging was that after the purpose had been achieved, God blessed the king.

I could also see that there was a definite reason that God took everything, including his mind, away from King Nebuchadnezzar. But in my case God's reasons were not quite so clear. I didn't believe that as in King Nebuchadnezzar's case, pride or not admitting that God was Lord, was the reason for my psychosis. But even though I couldn't see it right now, there still must be some purpose. I clung to that hope! My illness must also be a part of God's plan for my life. Although at that time I *felt* like saying "What have You done?" if I was to believe scripture then I knew that what God did, or allowed, was *right* and *just*.

I also did some studying in Job. I could relate to Job's trials that seemed to occur one after the other, and his depression. But the message that came out very clearly to me, was that God was in control. I might not understand what happened, but God still had His hand on the situation. Also there was an end to Job's suffering, as was the case with

King Nebuchadnezzar. There was a time of healing and restoration, a time when God gave back even more than was taken away. It was wonderfully reassuring to know that God was in control of my life, whatever might happen. I knew that God didn't allow me to get sick just to hurt me. Just as earthly fathers (mothers) hurt with their children as they are in pain, so God must feel the pain of His children. The big difference with God is He sees the larger picture. Even though *I* might not see the purpose now, God *could* see the end result.

As I continued to search my Bible, I came up with a couple of possible reasons for my illness to have happened to me.

> *"'Neither this man nor his parents sinned,' said Jesus, 'but this happened so that the work of God might be displayed in his life.' "* (John 9:3)

> *"Praise be to the God and Father of our Lord Jesus Christ, the Father of compassion and the God of all comfort, who comforts us in all our troubles, so that we can comfort those in any trouble with the comfort we ourselves have received from God."* (2 Corinthians 1:3-4)

I couldn't truthfully say that at that point I felt that God had given me comfort at all in the real sense. But I could see that He might possibly use what I had gone through to help others in similar situations. I still found it very difficult to understand how God could allow mental illness, particularly psychosis, but I knew it happened. For Christians to be somehow exempt would be not only unfair but also tragic. Non-Christians would have no hope. I cannot imagine going through the horror of a psychosis and feeling that it was just a random happening, that there is no one in control of your life but yourself. One of the most frightening things about a psychosis is that *you* are not in control. You can't control your emotions, your thoughts, or your actions. We humans like to feel that we are in control, that we can trust ourselves to survive. Well, after a psychosis, you realize that you cannot trust yourself in every circumstance. Therefore, you feel a desperate need to know that there is someone greater than you that you can trust, someone who is in control.

I not only searched the Bible for answers, I also looked for any information I could get—from books to TV—that would give me a better understanding of what I had been through. I found myself drawn to shows about manic-depression, schizophrenia, and even Alzheimer's disease. I found I could relate to different symptoms in each one of these illnesses. Through gaining a better understanding of them, I was able to understand more about my psychosis and depression.

I searched for and found a book, written from a Christian perspective, about dealing with physical suffering. It was a great book, if you were in physical pain, but it didn't even touch on emotional or mental suffering.

One day, out of boredom and a sense of isolation, I turned the TV on to "The Donahue Show." The panel of all women was sharing their personal experiences with postpartum depression and/or postpartum psychosis. Of course, being *The Donahue Show*, their stories were sensational, to say the least. One woman had shot herself in the stomach while pregnant, one had thrown her baby over the side of a bridge, and still another had drowned hers. The audience's reaction, quite understandably, ranged from horror and disbelief, to anger and disgust. On the opposite side, were my own feelings: understanding, pain, and a sense of anticipation. I might finally get some answers about Postpartum Depression and Psychosis. After listening to the panel of women explain their experiences I felt so fortunate that nothing equally tragic had happened in my case. It so easily could have. I could understand the thinking patterns which led these women to injure themselves or their baby. One woman had drowned her baby because she thought it was Satan. She felt her husband was Jesus Christ and would raise the baby from the dead again. I too had been afraid Martina might be possessed or that Kurt was possessed. I had also been sure that if I jumped out of a window I would be able to fly.

As I raptly watched the program, I was so grateful to God that I had not harmed anyone during my psychosis. That had been my greatest fear upon coming out of the psychosis, that I might have injured someone. The pain I was experiencing could be nothing compared to that of the mom who had killed her child! The show definitely gave me a better understanding of postpartum depression/psychosis and a more positive perspective. I may have suffered, but others had suffered even more.

Over the next several weeks I learned that different people in my church had suffered with mental illness—from manic-depression, to a psychosis during the onset of menopause. Those who had a psychotic episode completely recovered. Others doggedly persevered with a continuing illness. But in both cases, seeing what they were accomplishing with their lives really gave me hope. I also felt less alone.

Although I was no longer severely depressed, as while in hospital, I was still struggling. I would cry almost every day, not necessarily because I was sad, but the tears just seemed to flow. My energy level was also very low. I found it difficult to accomplish everyday tasks around home. Setting realistic goals and making *to do* lists for the day, week, etc.

really helped, not only to encourage me, but also because my short term memory was very poor. If I were asked what I had done the previous day, my mind would likely go completely blank.

When Kurt took the car to work, I was basically house bound. I did try to get out with Martina for a walk whenever I could. On occasion we would stop at the park to feed the ducks. Even when Kurt was home, it helped to go out for a walk, and talk about future plans, such as holidays we'd like to take together. Somehow getting out of the confining walls of the apartment seemed to remove me beyond the depression, so I could breathe easier and look ahead to the future.

I remember asking the psychiatrist at the Mental Health Center how long my depression would last. He gave me a very good answer: "Dorothy, your recovery from depression is going to be like growing hair. You don't see your hair growing day by day but a month down the road, when you need a trim, you realize, yes, it has grown. In the same way, you won't see yourself improving day by day but a month down the road when you look back to what you were like, you will see that, yes, you are feeling better."

I found my recovery just this way. From day to day, I didn't feeling any improvement, yet from month to month it was definitely measurable.

TWELVE

Fear, Nightmares, and the Word

What I found most difficult to deal with in my depression was my feelings of fear and anxiety. I had scary thoughts—almost pictures—in my head. An example would be when using a sharp knife, clearly seeing it cutting into my skin. Or when giving Martina a bath, seeing her head go under the water. Although I definitely would not have purposely cut myself, or allowed Martina's head to go under in the bath, these pictures just flashed through my mind. I later learned these *scary thoughts* were very common in postpartum depression. At that time, however, they terrified me.

Also on occasion when I'd glance in the mirror at my

reflection, usually when I was home alone, my own eyes would scare me. It was as if a stranger was looking back. It was the same feeling I had when, as a child, I watched a scary movie and was afraid of my own hands in bed that night. Often when I'd lie in bed at night with my eyes closed, strange images of horrible creatures would flash through my mind.

Nightmares were also a symptom of my depression during this time, not to mention the greatest cause of my fear and anxiety. If I would not get enough sleep or if I got up with Kurt early in the morning, then went back to bed, I would have terrifying dreams. It wasn't necessarily the content of the dream; it was the feeling of confusion and terror that went with it. I would often dream that I was psychotic again. Or other times, in my dream, I would wake up, see myself in bed awake, and then realize I was still sleeping. Once I saw an elusive figure cloaked in black standing by my bed. I would try desperately to wake up, to open my eyes, but I couldn't. My mind seemed half-asleep in the nightmare and yet half-awake. It was terribly frightening. I began to dread sleeping each night lest I have another nightmare.

The fear reached a peak one evening. Kurt was out of town; I felt alone and vulnerable. I got into bed that night with a terrible feeling of fear and anxiety inside. I felt a terrible smothering darkness threaten me, closing in on me.

On an impulse I picked up my Bible. I read through some Psalms that I had memorized years ago, but since my psychosis could not remember. These included:

Psalm 46 *"God is our refuge and strength, A very present help in trouble. Therefore we will not fear..."*

"Hear my cry, O God; Give heed to my prayer. From the end of the earth I call to Thee, when my heart is faint; Lead me to the rock that is higher than I. For Thou hast been a refuge for me, A tower of strength against the enemy, Let me dwell in Thy tent forever; Let me take refuge in the shelter of Thy wings." (Psalm 61:1-4)

"O God, Thou art my God; I shall seek Thee earnestly; ...When I remember Thee on my bed, I meditate on Thee in the night watches, For Thou hast been my help, And in the shadow of Thy wings I sing for joy. My soul clings to Thee; Thy right hand upholds me." (Psalm 63:1-8)

"...You will not be afraid of the terror by night...For He will give His angels charge concerning you, To guard you in all your

146

ways…Because he has loved Me, therefore I will deliver him; I will set him securely on high, because he has known My name. He will call upon Me, and I will answer him; I will be with him in trouble; I will rescue him, and honor him. With a long life I will satisfy him, And let him behold My salvation." (Psalm 91)

"I will lift up my eyes to the mountains; From whence shall my help come? My help comes from the Lord… The Lord is your keeper; The Lord is your shade on your right hand. The sun will not smite you by day, Nor the moon by night. The Lord will protect you from all evil; He will keep your soul…" (Psalm 121)

"…If I say, 'Surely the darkness will overwhelm me, And the light around me will be night,' Even the darkness is not dark to Thee, And the night is as bright as the day." (Psalm 139)

As I read these passages it felt like a dark cloud lifting. In place of anxiety there was a blanket of peace.

"Peace I leave with you; my peace I give you…Do not let your heart be troubled and do not be afraid…" "Do

not be anxious about anything, but in everything, by prayer and petition, with thanksgiving, present your requests to God. And the peace of God, which transcends all understanding, will guard your hearts and your minds in Christ Jesus."

I could scarcely believe how my fear and anxiety went away. That night I had a peaceful sleep with no nightmares. I cannot honestly say that I never felt any fear after that night but it was under control and not nearly as bad. I knew God could take it away and I had a very powerful tool to use against it—the Bible. Although I did very rarely still dream of being psychotic, which was naturally disturbing, I never again had the particularly disturbing nightmare where I fought to wake up.

Now I don't know for certain exactly what role Satan had in my dreams. I do know, however, that Satan attacks us where we are weakest. Well, after going through a psychosis, my mind was extremely vulnerable to fear and anxiety. In his book *Spiritual Warfare*, Timothy M. Warner says: "A demon charged with harassing me would be a fool to see me having an emotional or mental problem and not try to complicate it." What so encouraged me was that through God's Word I could put an end to such harassment.

After that night, when through God's Word I had victory over my fear and anxiety, I felt much closer to God. He had cared for me in such an extremely personal way. It fascinated and awed me that God knew all those years ago, when I was memorizing these particular passages, what I would go through and how they would help me. My Bible verses were the glue that held me together. Although it may have been God's plan for me to go through a psychosis and subsequent depression, living in a state of constant fear and anxiety was not what He wanted.

In March, I was given an increase in lithium, which also helped to improve my mood. I began to see how much I had to be thankful for. I had a terrific husband, a healthy, happy baby and I was slowly but surely improving. One day on the *Focus on the Family* radio program a woman shared her story of losing her baby to SIDS very shortly after giving birth. Even as I cried for her pain, I was so grateful for the gift of Martina. I had missed the first few months of her life, but I had her now, and God willing for many years to come.

That spring, my sister-in-law, Darlene, also came to visit. We had a chance to talk about my illness—what I experienced and also what she remembered. I limited the conversation to my symptoms during my psychosis, not even mentioning what the psychosis had done to me as a person, or about my depression. That was still a subject that was too close to me, too painful. The impression I wanted to give was that of a well person. So I had been psychotic, but I was through that and life could go on as normal.

By the time I was taken off lithium in June I was feeling a lot better. We were somewhat concerned I might have a relapse after being taken off medication but, if anything, I felt even better, more myself. My short-term memory was still poor, but I had heard other new moms complaining of the same problem.

As the months went by, as our family made new memories, my postpartum experience began to diminish in significance for me. It was no longer always in the back of my mind; I began living in the present and looking to the future instead of constantly reviewing the past.

On a few occasions, I did share with friends my experience; it was healing to do so. And it was freeing to realize that my sense of identity was no longer as inexorably tied up with my psychosis and subsequent depression as it once was.

THIRTEEN

New Beginnings

*I*n the spring of 1989, one year after being taken off lithium, our family moved to Edmonton, Alberta due to a job transfer. It was a big change for us; we had enjoyed living in Vancouver. Yet for myself, leaving the city where I had so many bad memories mixed with the good, was freeing. I was looking forward to life in a new city, along with a new beginning.

Edmonton was to bring greater changes than just a new home. After much thought, Kurt and I had decided to have another child. I got pregnant in 1990, three years after my previous pregnancy. My feelings regarding this pregnancy were mixed. I was no less happy and excited than when I was pregnant with Martina. But I also had to deal with the possibility of getting sick again. I remember going for a walk by myself and hashing everything through.

There was still this 1 in 3 chance of becoming psychotic again after the birth of the baby. For my part, I realized that there was absolutely nothing I could do to prevent it if another bout of postpartum psychosis was in God's plan for my life. I could just prepare myself as best I could for the eventuality and leave the rest in God's hands. Now, I did definitely pray that I would not get sick. But I also asked God to protect my family and myself in the event that postpartum psychosis occurred again.

Part of my preparing for another postpartum illness was making my new family doctor fully aware of my experience with postpartum psychosis. He was quite interested to know that lithium was what brought me out of the psychosis. According to him, this was significant because lithium also affected the thyroid gland. He felt it would be in my best interest to see a thyroid specialist during my pregnancy.

The thyroid specialist also felt that the affect lithium had on my psychosis was significant. Although he was not ready to say that my thyroid gland was definitely a cause of my previous illness, it was at least a possible link. Because pregnancy often affects the thyroid gland, he wanted my thyroxin level closely monitored. Over the period of nine months, my thyroxin level went down significantly. It was necessary for me to take twice as much thyroxin hormone than I regularly did.

There was also a slight possibility that I could get sick during the pregnancy as my hormones shifted, but I was fine. I did, however, have a dream one night that made me somewhat anxious. Now many people have frightening dreams. It does not mean that they are about to become psychotic. But as a general rule I'm not the type of person who has nightmares. And because of the frightening dreams that I had when first becoming ill, this particular dream rang an alarm bell inside me. It was very similar to the ones I had while in the hospital directly following Martina's birth. Again, although the dream was not that frightening by itself, the feeling inside of me was stark fear. In the dream, Kurt and I were driving by an accident site. We watched as a man came out of the wrecked car. Before our eyes, he became hideously deformed. At that point I had that all too familiar feeling of terror and woke suddenly.

In the morning I told Kurt about my dream. He was his usual calm and sensible self. "Dorothy," he assured me, "It's just one dream. It probably meant nothing."

As he predicted, there were no more frightening dreams. I slept very well throughout the rest of my pregnancy. Because I dealt with the fear of getting sick again at the beginning of my pregnancy, I didn't feel the need nor have the desire to dwell on it through the remaining months. There would be time enough to worry after the baby was born. Now I wanted to concentrate on this special little life I was carrying and prepare for him/her as best I could.

Aside from a sore back my pregnancy went very smoothly. I felt great physically, emotionally, and mentally. The months flew by as I cared for Martina, busied myself inside the house and also outside in the garden. Many evening hours were spent knitting tiny sweaters, hats, and booties. This was a very special time for me; after having one difficult postpartum period I no longer took good health,— physical, emotional, or mental, for granted.

Like many husbands, Kurt waited until after the baby was born to get outwardly excited. But there was one little individual in our home who just couldn't wait. Martina had always loved babies, since she was just one year old. Her mothering instinct was very strong and I think she was looking forward to the arrival of a baby almost as much as I was. Throughout the pregnancy, Martina paged tirelessly through books showing the stages of a baby's growth inside the mother's womb, all the while asking me many questions. While grocery shopping, she would frequently ask any woman she met: "Do you have a baby in your tummy too?" It was very sweet. The women were not at all offended although most of them were not even pregnant.

I tried to physically prepare for the baby's birth in every possible way. The freezer was filled with a month worth of meals, complete with half a dozen apple pies and cookies. I didn't want to worry about cooking after the baby was born. I just wanted to relax and enjoy the special time that I had missed after the birth of Martina. I had also arranged for my mother to pick Martina up and take her home to Prince George following the birth of the new baby. Not only did I want to be able to concentrate on caring for the baby, but also in case I got sick I felt it would be better if Martina was out of the way.

The baby's due date was October 28. Because I had been induced before Martina was born, I didn't really know what to expect this time. I really didn't want to be overdue again. As it turned out I went into labour one day early. We arrived in hospital around seven p.m. and before midnight we had another beautiful daughter, Natasha Alexis.

Yes, it was just as special the second time around. And because my labour was short with no complications afterward, my physical recovery was surprisingly quick. Within a couple hours of the delivery, I was able to enjoy a large supper. Natasha was kept in the nursery for the first night to allow me at least one good night's rest.

In the morning, it was time to adjust to a newborn again. It amazed me that two babies from the same family could look so different yet be so uniquely special. Whereas

Martina had been born with a full head of hair, Natasha, although far from bald, had very little. It didn't take long for this new little one, who frowned just like her Dad, to worm her way deep into my heart.

When Martina came to the hospital that day to see her new baby sister, she was very delighted, exclaiming how *cute* and *tiny* Natasha was. She proudly held her; in fact, between Martina and Grandma, poor Dad hardly got a chance. After the visit, Martina left to go home with Grandma.

You could say I was my own psychiatrist the first days and even weeks after Natasha was born. I analyzed my every thought and feeling to see if it was *normal*. There was definitely an underlying fear and dread lest I get sick again. Yet on the surface I felt quite positive, taking things from day to day.

I had requested that a psychiatrist come to my room to talk with me while I was in hospital so we would get to know each other a bit in case I did get sick. As it turned out the psychiatrist sent his resident.

She had absolutely no warmth or bedside manner whatsoever. She just breezed into my hospital room and started firing questions at me. There I was, slightly flustered, trying to get used to breastfeeding a baby again. She didn't ask if this might be a bad time, how the baby was doing, nothing. In fact, she took no notice of Natasha whatsoever. She just started right in with very personal questions—about the last time I was sick, my background, and my marriage. All this she asked without any sense that she cared at all. It was obvious to me that she was trying to find a psychological reason for my prior illness, or possibly to rule it out.

I felt outraged and resented being put in such a position but didn't dare show it. After all, I needed to appear *normal*. Anyone else could have and no doubt would have asked her to leave, or come back after the baby had nursed, but I didn't feel in a position to do that. I was on the defensive, and I felt threatened. I could understand that since she didn't have the details of my illness she needed to ask certain questions to rule out psychological causes. But she could have done it in a much more acceptable way. Doctors and nurses had questioned me before; it wasn't the questions that bothered me. It was the lack of caring. She acted as though I was not even a real person.

The psychiatrist came himself the next day. After seeing his intern I really didn't know what to expect but I was pleasantly surprised. "Well, your previous psychosis was obviously caused by a chemical imbalance," he commented in a very friendly manner. "If you start showing signs of becoming ill, we'll put you on lithium right away."

I felt reassured as the doctor spoke of the facilities in the hospital where I could care for Natasha even if I became sick. Or if I was too ill, at least visit her often. I had prepared myself for a separation from Natasha if necessary, but knowing I could see her even if I got sick was great. This doctor's confident and matter of fact tone was very comforting and encouraging to me. I had expected to have to stay in hospital at least a week to see whether I would get sick or not. However, the doctor felt I might as well go home since my illness would not necessarily show up by then, if I were even to get sick this time. At the first sign of symptoms I could come back to hospital.

I felt certain that I could recognize another psychotic episode coming, as I did have some symptoms before actually becoming psychotic. Both Kurt and I would be on the lookout for extreme talkativeness, euphoria, and mania, not to mention any other unusual behaviour.

I was let out of hospital after the usual three days. On the way home, we went shopping to get a few things. I remember feeling slightly disorientated at the store. Was this normal after staying a few days in hospital?

Aside from the underlying fear of myself getting sick, I had a wonderful first few days at home with Natasha. It was like God gave me back the time I missed before. I so enjoyed looking after my newborn, although I did miss Martina terribly. Talking to her on the phone at Grandma's made me really struggle with tears. Somehow I hadn't expected to miss her quite so much.

Natasha was a very good baby although she had a tendency to want to drink all night for a while. Because I had prepared meals before the baby was born, Kurt and I could really take it easy and relax. We had our frozen meals, complete with apple pie or cookies for dessert; it was wonderful. In a sense, it was like before we had kids. I found a newborn much less work than an active 3-year-old who talked almost non-stop. Kurt also had several days off work to help me look after the baby and basically keep me company. So in the evenings Kurt and I could just sit together and talk, or watch TV.

Although I did not feel as if I was getting sick, I did experience some euphoria. Life just seemed to have an added zest to it. TV seemed more vivid, and I was excited about the future. This concerned me somewhat but I tried to keep in mind my psychiatrist's words: "Euphoria is actually very common in postpartum women. That alone, is not a cause to worry." So, as the days passed, with no additional symptoms, I began to relax. I did have a curious sense of déjà vu the first time I went to a store by myself after Natasha was born. Might I get lost again? But no, I made it home without incident. I did feel some disorientation, but I finally realized this too, like euphoria, might also be a *normal* postpartum feeling. I had been so afraid to have any of the same feelings I had following Martina's birth. To me they were all linked with the psychosis. It greatly reassured me to know that I could feel euphoric, overly emotional, disorientated, and even have the odd strange dream due to lack of sleep, without having to fear a mental breakdown.

FOURTEEN

Emotional Healing

As each day passed, my fear of becoming sick again decreased just a little more. Often while lying in bed at night I would find myself reviewing my whole experience with postpartum psychosis. It was no longer quite as painful to think about now that the threat was not so great. I was so very thankful for my health and wondered how I might use my experience with postpartum psychosis to help others, perhaps even form a support group? I was open to God's leading, but I fully realized that with a busy preschooler and a new baby, the timing might not be right.

When Martina came home from Grandma and Grandpa's, our family was complete. Martina was just bursting with energy and excitement over her new baby sister, Natasha. She liked to hold her; in fact, her technique was better than many adults. While I nursed Natasha, Martina would often hold her favourite teddy bear close, pretending to also be nursing. I loved watching the two of them interact; it was an extra special part of having two children.

As time went on, I became immersed in my growing family. To me, my postpartum illness was safely behind me. It could no longer *hurt* me. Yet, time and emotional distance did not necessarily remove the pain. I found that the emotions were always very close to the surface when I discussed my past illness with anyone.

I didn't recognize and truly deal with these emotions until several months later. Our family had been invited to a pastor friend of ours, actually the same pastor who had married us some eight years earlier. During the course of conversation, my experience with postpartum psychosis was mentioned along with my desire to possibly start a support group.

Pastor Morris listened intently, and then asked me some very direct questions: "Through starting a support group would you hope to get support yourself?" That one shook up my composure somewhat. What really did me in was his next question, "Dorothy, do you feel that you still have scars inside from going through the psychosis?"

That simple question tore me apart inside, revealing a great amount of pain and anger I had not even realized existed. Pain for the lost time with my baby that could never be regained, the horror of actually being psychotic, and intense hurt and anger for not having anyone who could understand. These feelings erupted in a fountain of healing tears.

That I still had these emotions and especially their intensity surprised me. It was like a dam being let loose. As we drove home that night I was still struggling not to cry, and I cried on and off for days. But it was a healing time for me. I realized it was all right for me to grieve; in fact it was necessary in order for me to heal completely.

I felt much better after dealing with these feelings. I assumed mistakenly that now I had dealt with them all. But God showed me one more big one that I needed to acknowledge.

A special speaker, Jay Carty, presented his *Counter Attack* workshop at our church. One evening he was speaking on anger. I thought, 'Well, I've dealt with any anger I may have felt. That's not a problem for me anymore.'

But at the end of the service he said something that just seemed to hit me over the head...hard: "Some of you are angry at God. You're asking 'How could You let this happen? And it's really hard to admit that you're angry with God, but you're just not sure you can trust Him anymore."

I had never really thought about it before but that's exactly how I felt. I still couldn't understand how God could let anyone go through a psychosis—to be completely out of control—and if God could allow something so awful to happen to me, I didn't know if I could trust Him not to allow something even worse.

I broke down in tears once again. I realized how crucial trust in God was. Without it I had no true *faith*, just religious beliefs based on fear. I couldn't have a personal relationship with a Heavenly Father who I was afraid would whack me over the head whenever it suited Him to do so.

At home that night, I admitted to God my anger, my fear of trusting Him. I realized that I had been picturing God somewhat like my earthly father. My Dad was never big on words; he liked to show his love through giving gifts. So when God gave me the opposite of a gift, a severe trial, I saw that as a punishment. I knew the Bible was full of God's *words* of love to me; I needed to accept *them* and not measure God's love for me by circumstances in my life.

I finally had to just say to God: "O.K., so I don't understand; I probably never will. That doesn't really matter. I *will* trust you! I know you love me, and whatever you allow to happen to me is according to your plan. You will give me the strength to go through it and the opportunity to use it for good."

So, I could trust God, not necessarily to keep me safe

from physical, emotional, financial, or even mental problems, but to keep my soul safe.

I had a real sense of healing after that night, like I had finally cleaned out my emotional closet. And things were different. When Pastor Morris and his wife came over to visit I was able to share with them more about my psychosis and what God had been teaching me, all without tears. I would always feel some pain about my experience with postpartum psychosis, but the wounds were healing, and no longer infecting the rest of my life.

As I completed the rough draft of this manuscript I happened to be memorizing Romans 5:1-11, which was amazingly appropriate, especially verses 3-5.

> *"Not only so, but we also rejoice in our sufferings, because we know that suffering produces perseverance; perseverance, character; and character, hope. And hope does not disappoint us, because God has poured out his love into our hearts by the Holy Spirit, whom he has given us."*

EPILOGUE

From Shattered Dreams

*F*ive years following the birth of Natasha, Kurt and I had yet another special baby, our third daughter, Sonja Nicole. Thankfully, I once again had a very *normal* postpartum period!

Now looking back, I realize how very blessed I am. I have three beautiful, healthy daughters—a definite blessing, but more than that, I can now see my whole experience with postpartum psychosis as a blessing, although admittedly still a painful one.

I have gained a new understanding and empathy for people who suffer from depression and other mental illnesses. In 3 short months I had a crash course in understanding basically all of the symptoms involved in most mental illnesses. I wouldn't choose to have that understanding; nevertheless I do. And because of the time that has passed, including 2 more pregnancies with no repeat of the psychosis or depression, I now feel distanced and *safe* enough emotionally to support others.

Just before Sonja was born, our family made another move, this time to Calgary, AB. Since then God has clearly directed me in helping others experiencing postpartum depression/psychosis. It has been so rewarding to be involved as a volunteer for new mothers experiencing postpartum depression. Hearing them say, "I don't know what I would have done if I didn't have you to talk to..." is worth so much. I have also had the privilege to share my postpartum experience with health care workers at a conference on Postpartum Mood Disorders.

I don't know what God has planned for my future, but I am confident He will continue to use my experience with postpartum psychosis to help others. So, although going through postpartum psychosis and its subsequent depression was the most frightening, painful, and difficult time of my life, it was also the most character building. I certainly would never want to go through it again, but looking at it from the other side, I can honestly say it was a gift! I can certainly agree in my heart with this verse:

*"In Him we were also chosen, having been predestined according to the plan of him who works out **everything** in conformity with the purpose of His will..."* (Ephesians 1:11)

APPENDIX ONE

Getting the Support You Need

If you have recently experienced postpartum psychosis (PPP) or depression (PPD), my primary advice to you is: Get whatever help and support you need. Find someone you can trust to help you to work through your experience and unresolved feelings. I was shocked recently, when reading some accounts of women who have suffered through postpartum psychosis and depression, that they had not shared their experience with anyone until much time had gone by. It may be a trusted friend, or a counsellor, but find someone to talk to. Or find many *someones*. For myself, although I never was able to talk to anyone who had also gone through postpartum psychosis, there were many people, family and friends, whose listening ear and support were invaluable. Not one individual could give me the support I needed. But together, they were able, through their patient listening and not judging, to help me along the road to healing.

Also, writing about your feelings and what you have experienced is also therapeutic. It allows you to distance yourself from them. Don't give up if you are at first not happy with the support you receive. When Kurt first contacted a postpartum support group, he was told that postpartum depression was caused by the pressures society put on women. This was, obviously, not very helpful. But I believe there is much more accurate information and available support now, for those touched by postpartum depression and psychosis.

Especially if you have had postpartum psychosis, it may be difficult for you to find someone who can understand you, even in a postpartum depression support group. You might want to do a search on the internet for what is available in your area. At the two following websites you will find a wealth of information and support, as well as listings of support groups.

postpartumprogress.typepad.com

postpartum.net

Also, an excellent book to read for more information on postpartum psychosis specifically is Teresa M. Twomey's book, *Understanding Postpartum Psychosis – A Temporary Madness*. It has the most current information, as well as sharing several women's personal stories.

Just a word of caution for those who have experienced postpartum psychosis, and wish greater understanding through reading the stories of other mothers with PPP. Proceed slowly, and carefully. When I experienced postpartum psychosis in 1987, there was hardly any information available. The only time PPP was mentioned was when a new mother with PPP killed herself, or her baby, even though this happens only a small fraction of the time. The potential is still there. And each time, I would feel their pain, and realize what could have happened. Now, over 20 years later, there is much more available information and support through reading of other's experiences. And that is wonderful and needed. But guard yourself against taking on too much *pain* from other's experiences. Set healthy boundaries. I was, frankly, very surprised when I began to investigate the available material on postpartum psychosis, just how powerfully I felt the grief and pain of these courageous young women who had struggled through PPP. The *monster* –psychosis, with its fear, seemed once again so near. And my experience with PPP was over twenty years ago. So, pace yourself, and possibly debrief with your spouse or a trusted friend.

When I made the decision to publish my story, God seemed to give me a word of caution as well, to go back to my past experiences to be able to support others, but not to *live* there. To keep moving *forward* in my healing to what God has for me in the future. So that is my prayer for you as well, that although you may need to process your experiences with PPP and PPD, you will not stay in the past, allowing it to paralyze you, but that you would use it to propel you forward, into the future that God has for you.

APPENDIX TWO

A Husband's Experience

by Kurt Ruhwald

Initially, when Dorothy started showing signs of disorientation and confusion, I really didn't know whether to take her symptoms very seriously or not. I didn't know what *normal* postpartum behaviour was and what wasn't. I also had no idea of how far this could go or how serious this was. Dorothy was exhibiting excited behaviour that seemed like it could be normal, even though it wasn't usual for her. However, when she *lost* the car I became very concerned, but I was still optimistic that Dorothy would get over whatever was bothering her, and would just get better. Soon after that, though, Dorothy's condition deteriorated very rapidly and my anxiety and stress level increased just as rapidly.

For a short time, Dorothy had some lucid moments in which she described what was happening to her. Her fear left me feeling powerless to protect her… I couldn't fix this, and I didn't know what to do.

Dorothy soon became un-manageable and needed supervision 24 hours a day: Dorothy throwing things into the tub, walking up to a floor to ceiling window muttering about flying, and taking the scissors and trying to cut the cords that controlled the blinds made that point clear. Dealing with Dorothy, my new job, and caring for baby Martina became just too much for both Dorothy's mother, who was staying with us for a week, and for me. We needed help.

It's strange how these sorts of things tend to happen just at the start of a holiday long weekend, but we were able to see our family doctor before he left for the weekend. Luckily, he had been able to get to know Dorothy over the past several months and I feel this made it easier for him to recognize the state Dorothy was in. He made the arrangements for Dorothy to be hospitalized if necessary during the weekend and he gave me instructions on where to take Dorothy if she didn't improve and if I couldn't cope anymore. Well, that point had already passed, but I was willing to see how Dorothy would do over the weekend. Well, Dorothy did not improve. She got worse, so I decided to hospitalize her. This was not a decision that I had to agonize over; it was obvious to me and I had no doubts; she was a risk to herself, to her baby and to those around her. While taking Dorothy to the hospital, she was completely catatonic although she could walk with my guidance. Dorothy needed round the clock supervision in a safe and secure environment that I could not provide.

During the next few days, I needed a break; I spent some time with my cousin and friend. I went hiking and chopped some wood, which I found was very therapeutic. I also needed rest; I was exhausted. My mother-in-law went back home; she was also exhausted. Baby Martina went to be with my parents. I was lucky to have a support network of family and friends to care for my needs and those of Martina. This was very important to my wellbeing; I owe them a lot for that period of time.

I was able to keep on working, but in hindsight it would have been better if I had taken a leave of absence. I was juggling work, with visiting Dorothy and caring for Martina on my days off. I soon realized that Dorothy did not seem to be aware of the passage of time and I concluded that I would run myself ragged if I tried to visit Dorothy every day. Since she wouldn't be aware that I had missed a day or two, I started coming in to visit her only on my days off. This helped to relieve my fatigue level but I was still under a lot of stress.

Dorothy had changed; all aspects of her personality had changed so much that I no longer knew her. I had no idea when Dorothy would come out of her psychosis, or even if she ever would. My life was in a state of limbo. I thought, *"What if she never came out of it...?"* The situation was worse than if she would have bled out and died while giving birth to Martina. My wife was gone, yet she was still alive. Even so, I believed that somewhere inside her, the real Dorothy was still there—trapped and very scared; I wasn't going to give up.

In general, I found that the health care providers that were caring for Dorothy were very good – professional and compassionate. There were, however, those that insisted that Dorothy take some responsibility in the ward. One of those responsibilities would be caring for her own clothing and personal care. The outcome was that while in the hospital, Dorothy lost numerous articles of clothing including a house coat that I gave her as a wedding present and her wedding rings. We didn't discover this until after Dorothy came out of the psychosis – too late to recover anything. Dorothy also wore the same pair of contact lenses for weeks without removing them at night or cleaning them – this could have done lasting damage to her eyes, but went un-discovered or un-remedied by the caregivers.

I thought that the whole idea of treating a sick mind by expecting its exercise made about as much sense as telling someone with a broken leg to walk on it without a cast until it feels better. This method of treatment frustrated me and it reduced my confidence in the caregivers. I thought they just didn't understand; Dorothy was gone and couldn't be responsible for anything. I thought that if they would only have known Dorothy before she got sick then they would understand how far gone she was and how futile their attempts to reason with her were. I couldn't get through to Dorothy, so how did they expect to? I still feel it was the caregivers' fault that Dorothy lost her personal possessions.

I am also convinced that women who suffered a postpartum psychosis like Dorothy, but were unfortunately not prevented from harming their own babies or loved ones, should not be incarcerated. They do not need punishment; they need care and compassion, and they need to be told it was not their fault. Because once they come out of their psychosis, and realize that their babies are gone by their own hands, they will be inconsolable.